THE HUMAN TESTIS: A CLINICAL TREATISE

THE HUMAN TESTIS: A CLINICAL TREATISE

By

LEONARD PAUL WERSHUB, M.D., F.A.C.S., F.I.C.S.

Diplomate of American Board of Urology
Associate Professor of Urology
New York Medical College
Metropolitan Medical Center
New York City

With Forewords by

Ralph E. Snyder, M.D.
New York Medical College

and

Charles Montgomery Stewart, M.D.
University of Southern California Medical School

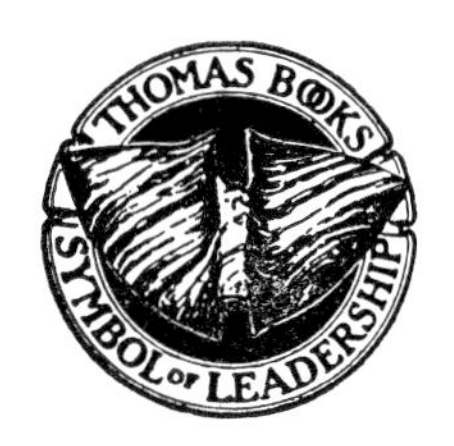

CHARLES C THOMAS • PUBLISHER
Springfield • Illinois • U.S.A.

CHARLES C THOMAS • PUBLISHER

BANNERSTONE HOUSE

301-327 East Lawrence Avenue, Springfield, Illinois, U.S.A.

Library of Congress Catalog Card Number: 61-13449

With THOMAS BOOKS careful attention is given to all details of manufacturing and design. It is the Publisher's desire to present books that are satisfactory as to their physical qualities and artistic possibilities and appropriate for their particular use. THOMAS BOOKS will be true to those laws of quality that assure a good name and good will.

Printed in the United States of America

To

Hyman Jordan Sobiloff

Semper Amicus

"There are many problems and difficulties in the education of a medical student, but they are not more difficult than the question of the continuous education of the general practitioner . . . No class of men needs to call to mind more often the wise comment of Plato that education is a life-long business."

WILLIAM OSLER

FOREWORD

Since the dark, dim pages of man's past, the mysteries of the testes have assumed a predominant role in the preoccupation of human thought. The symbolism of the testes and its many meanings interwoven through the sketchily recorded history of man is eloquent testimony of man's search for deeper knowledge and understanding of human function.

The search for knowledge in medicine has slowly pushed back the barriers to understanding and the shadows of superstition surrounding the testes. Indeed, it is only within recent history that the dawn of true understanding of the functions and importance of the testes have occurred. The development of laboratory research and biochemical techniques have opened many new, heretofore unknown and unrecognized functional roles.

That the knowledge of the function of the testes spans many disciplines in our highly specialized profession is now recognized. This knowledge is now an integral part of the knowledge of all medicine. It is fitting, proper and timely that this knowledge should be gathered in a single volume for the continuing education of medical students and all practitioners of medicine, whether specialists or not. The continued growth of medical knowledge and its dissemination depends upon the addition of intelligent, understandable and yet scholarly scientific contributions to that of our recorded knowledge.

Ralph E. Snyder, M.D.
President and Dean
New York Medical College
Flower and Fifth Avenue Hospitals
New York City

FOREWORD

SHAKESPEARE once said, "To hold as it 'twere the mirror up to nature." This statement might alert us not to believe that it was by mere chance that the lovliest and most treasured flower that grows and the male gonad should have the same name. The poetico-mystical-mythologic-philosophic-historical backround of this close relationship in nomenclature is worthy of recording in the foreword to this monumental scientific text.

The Greek term orchis, meaning testes, provided Theophrastus, the renouned philospher and student of Plato and Aristotle, with the word-root for the botanical term orchid, which he originated to designate a genus of plants peculiar to the Mediterranean regions. The first appearance of the word "orchis" was in his Greek Manuscript titled, "Enquiry into Plants" written sometime between 370-285 B.C. He is referred to as the "Father of Botany" or the "Father of Orchidology."

Theophrastus probably originated the term orchid from orchis, in allusion to what he believed to be a fancied similarity between the paired, enlarged, underground bulbs of the plant and the testicles of humans which were commonly described as being, "a pair of fleshy tuberoids."

In the history of orchid appreciation, the Oriental influence long antedated that in Europe as is evidenced by a quotation from Confucius (551-479 B.C.) that "acquaintance with good men was like entering a room full of lan, or fragrant orchids."

According to the Doctrine of Signatures, which flourished during the Middle Ages, the predestined use of a plant was indicated by its form. So it is interesting that Dioscorides, who dominated the botanical thought for sixteen centuries during the Middle Ages, considered orchis roots as influencing sexual phenomena. Specifically, an infusion of the younger and firmer of these two "bulbs" was believed to stimulate production of a male child and that made from the older and softer ones was thought to incite production of a female child.

Orchids provided the source for many herbal medicaments. The Bodianus Manuscript, an Aztec herbal writing of 1552, records the earliest reference to the use of orchid herbal extracts for this purpose. It is interesting to note that vanilla, an extract of the orchid (genus vanilla) was widely used in the concoction of various juices to produce a "lotion to be used against fatigue of those holding public office." It was recorded that this lotion was thought to "bestow the bodily strength of a gladiator; drive weariness far away and finally drive out fear and fortify the human heart."

In 1665 the German Jesuit Athanasius Kircher, in his Mundus Subterraneous, noted that orchids or "Satyria" sprang up, in places where the animals were brought together for breeding, through the escape upon the ground of spermatic fluid. For this reason these plants were thought to stimulate lust.

Living things possess three basic capacities, growth, adaption and reproduction. It is incomprehensible that scientific investigation of the reproductive function has been the last and the least studied of these three cardinal characteristics of living matter. Neither scientific honesty nor basic human dignity can be properly served with continued intellectual subserviency of the most dominating instinct of the human male animal: the urge and impulse of sex.

For those who prefer to believe that an understanding of life cannot be factually explained on the basis of evolution and who accept our world as the end result of a special creation—possibly they may deal more tolerantly with human weakness when they realize that insects and/or flowering plants have been found guilty of moral obliquity.

That the Greeks chose the name orchid from the word-root orchis, to permanently designate and classify this group of the world's most awe-inspiring floral masterpieces may not be as fanciful, tralatitious, mythical, whimsical or unpremeditated as one might think.

In 1862 Charles Darwin's classic treatise on the relation between insects and orchids was published. He banished all doubt regarding the function of pollen and centered attention on a complex symbiosis existing between orchids and food-seeking insects.

In 1916 Monsieur Pouyanne published the first series of articles with conclusions so startling that painstaking confirmation, during a period of twenty years, preceded their publication. Pouyanne had observed that flowers of the orchid Ophrys speculum are visited not only by a single species of insect (Scolis Dielis) but solely by the males of this species. He reported that the flowering season of Ophrys speculum coincides with the emerging of the male Scolia Ciliata from their burrows deep within the sun bathed banks of Algeria. The males emerge from their burrows about a month earlier than the females of the species. It is during this long wait for the appearance of the females, that the male insects visit the orchid flowers, finding in them a compelling attraction.

Pouyanne proved that the flowers of Ophrys speculum are not visited for nectar or edible tissues because when the males of Scolia Ciliata enter this flower the suctorial apparatus is not used and the insect's proboscis does not come in sustained contact with any part of the labellum of the orchid. The insects insert the tip of the abdomen rather than its head among the hairs of the orchid's labellum and the ensuing action of the insect is described as follows, "Le bout de l'abdomen est alors agité, contre ces poils, de mouvements désordonnes, presque convulsifs, et l'insecte tout entier se trémousse; ses mouvements, son attitude paraissent tout à fait semblables, à ceux des insectes que pratiquent des tentatives de copulation."

This orchid, it is believed, has an odor too faint for perception by human nostrils because this variety of orchid is described botanically as being without scent. Pouyanne said that there is a resemblance between the female of Scolia Ciliata and the labellum of the orchid, though inaccurate enough not to deceive the human eye, neverthless, possessing a sufficient degree of similarity to appear genuine to the known myopic vision peculiar to insects. He is convinced that a subtle scent is evident that completes the hoax and is responsible for induction of the sexual phenomena he so convincingly described.

Pouyanne's irrefutable experiments demonstrate that the behavior of the insects definitely proves a biologically adjusted and mutually advantageous reproductive symbiosis between Ophrys speculum and males of Scolia Ciliata. If these symbiotic purposes are purely sexual and this fact Pouyanne's observations and experiments have proved beyond a doubt, then the beauteous orchid alone has been biologically benefited by this association and we are forced to surmise, judging by human standards, that the Algerian insect has been sadly hoodwinked sexually.

With this background of factual, Grecian, biological and botanical, sexual phantasy concerning the loveliest of all of creation's flowers, it is most difficult to gracefully accept the following definition of "Testicle" from Taber's Cyclopedic Medical Dictionary; "one of two ovoid male gonads situated in the scrotum, which produce spermatozoa and some of the fluid elements of semen. They contain numerous secreting tubules in which the spermatozoa are produced, which are gathered from the Corpus of Highmore and ejected through the vas deferans. The testicles are suspended from the spermatic cords. The left one is lower than the right one."

How can it be possible to accept this casual, coldly definitive and deliberately impersonal description of the only corporal accoutrements essential to a man being a male and a male being a man?

Doctor Wershub's text is as comprehensive a record of the normalities and abnormalities of the development, structure and function of the human testes from conception to senescence as the foregoing discussion is genitally and endocrinologically irrelevant.

His profound contribution sharply magnifies the complicated, inseparable inter-dependance of the prime male genital unit and the endocrine system. It is a total summation of all of the substantiated facts and the theoretical considerations of the present day conception of urologic-endocrinology.

Each major facet of the subject is clearly discussed and the subject material of each chapter is finally summarized in brief outline for ready reference. The detailed discussions, followed by a concluding reference outline qualify this book as a readily understandable reference for medical students, urological resident physicians, practicing urologists, endocrinologists, general practioners, and for all physicians with special interests in the basic aspects of male fertility.

That Leonard Paul Wershub should be responsible for this currently complete, concise, meticulous, factual and theoretical contribution to Urology and Endocrinology was predestined. Doctor Wershub's previous scientific writings are incontestable evidence of his singular, lucid, communicable capacities as a medical littérateur. His completed text is as painstaking as it is titanic. It is a rare privilege to commend this erudite work to all urologists and endocrinologists as a permanent reference authority to be placed in their personal medical libraries.

Charles Montgomery Stewart, M.D.
Clinical Professor of Urology
University of Southern California
Medical School
Los Angeles, California

AUTHOR'S PREFACE

Within the past decade considerable contributions of an endocrinological nature have been added to the ever growing armamentarium of the urologist. A correlation of this new data is herewith presented in as concise a manner as is possible without the omission of pertinent data. Although the text as its title implies, is directed to testicular disturbances, I have deliberately avoided inflammatory disorders and specific infections of the testicle as well as other pathological processes of the testicle and its appendages. Such information is readily available in all standard text books of urology. Instead I have confined the text to testicular endocrinopathies. I have also included a discussion of the androgenital syndrome because of the intimate relationship between the adrenals and the testes. A chapter has been devoted to testicular tumors because of the endocrine factors in many of these neoplasms.

I fully realize that during the preparation and after the publication of this book, new and astounding revelations of an endocrine nature could and will be made. This book is herewith presented with facts and theories. It is my hope that it will serve as an aid in the clinical application of testicular endocrinopathies, and as a stimulus for the student interested in this field of clinical medicine, based of course on the data now available.

I wish to thank Doctor Paul M. Read for his constructive criticism of the original manuscript. I also wish to thank Doctor George Nagamatsu, Chairman of the Department of Urology, and the members of the staff whose cooperation was so essential for the compilation of this manuscript. Thanks are also due to Doctor Robert Blankfein for his aid in reading and rereading proofs. Finally, I wish to thank my secretary, Miss Joan Switzer, for her hours of difficult and meticulous labor in the never ending task of typing the final manuscript.

Leonard Paul Wershub

New York, N.Y.

CONTENTS

ILLUSTRATIONS

THE HUMAN TESTIS: A CLINICAL TREATISE

Chapter 1

INTRODUCTION

THE PRIMARY intent of this book is to present the modern concept of the biology of the human testes, with the hope that such a text will be of help to the physician who is confronted with the problems of testicular endocrinopathies. Although I have approached the subject from a urologist's point of view, the book is primarily written for the student and physician interested in this subject.

The past half century has witnessed tremendous research activity in the clinical phases of the endocrine system. The endocrinologist has contributed a vast new literature and a wealth of knowledge. Despite this great surge of information there has been a lack of correlation between the endocrinologist and the clinician. Since many of these endocrinopathic disorders involve the genitourinary system it seems only natural that greater cooperation should exist between the urologist and endocrinologist.

The efforts of researchers in endocrinology have resulted in an accumulation of data which has led to our present concept of *urologic endocrinology*. Such a broad classification of a vital subject does not necessarily exclude from this important phase of medicine the experimental embryologist, the physiologist, steroid chemist, internist and endocrinologist, biogeneticist, pediatrician and general practitioner, but, on the contrary, places emphasis upon their role in the recognition and management of these cases. Modern concepts of urologic endocrinology, plus the ever rapid growth of the medical literature on these subjects passes a heavy burden on to the urologist, calling upon him to keep posted with the rapid changes in thought and concept in the field of endocrinology.

It seems natural that patients, because of testicular derangement and testicular endocrinopathies, be referred to the urologist for specific urologic investigation. For this reason, the responsibility to recognize and understand the different symptoms, complexes and syndromes now included in the field of urologic endocrinology passes on to the urologist. For instance, virilism or hypogonadism may be the result of a pathologic process outside of the scrotal area, but with definite testicular derangement. Regardless of the etiologic factor, the urologist must be qualified to interpret and evaluate such disorders.

Since a testicular disturbance may be due to a disturbance of some endocrine gland, other than the testicle, it becomes even more important for the urologist to be familiar with the overall endocrine picture of the human male. Even though the text is confined to the biology of the testicle, it is difficult, if not impossible, to discuss only the problems of testicular endocrine disorders and avoid a consideration of the hypophyseal-pituitary adrenal-gonad axis.

In this presentation the author has not followed any specific outline of classification, but has tried instead to stress the urologic aspects of testicular endocrine problems, plus the adrenal and pituitary influences which so often overlap the clinical evaluation.

The physician with a diagnostic problem involving hormonal disturbances as evidenced by virilization and changes in growth and development now finds himself confronted with an embarrassing array of hormonal tests of testicular, adrenal or pituitary function. In many instances, a better understanding of these tests might eliminate unnecessary and expensive laboratory procedures in the search to determine the underlying cause of the clinical problem.

In the twenty-two years since the first adrenal steroid was isolated, twenty-nine compounds have been identified. Many clinicians divide the tests of adrenocortical function into two types: (1) direct tests in which by chemical means or by bioassay the amount of adrenal hormones are calculated as circulating in the blood or excreted in the urine; and (2) indirect tests in which an evaluation is made of the alterations in the blood and/or urine, produced by these hormones.

It follows that the direct tests are more expensive and are not always available, since they require special techniques mainly found in specialized steroid laboratories. Thus the indirect tests, particularly in conjunction with ACTH stimulation, are of great clinical value.

The recognition of the adreno-genital syndrome as a definite entity is now accepted as is the value of hormonal therapy in certain selected cases. It now becomes necessary for the physician to be familiar with the clinical picture of formerly supposed rare disorders, such as: female pseudohermaphroditism; macrogenitosomia praecox; adrenal virilism; and feminizing tumors in the male. Such diagnostic acumen has only recently been made possible by a better understanding of laboratory data, associated with physical findings and, in many instances, by accurate histologic interpretation made possible by testicular biopsy.

The recent advances in surgery of the adrenal glands, a glandular structure well within the realm of the urologic surgeon, have been made possible only by the corresponding advancements made in the physiology, hormonal investigations, biochemistry and pathology of this structure. But, what has been even more progressive, is the assay and development of potent extracts so essential for substitution therapy, in operations on the adrenal gland.

The significance of hormones and neoplastic disease has been of great interest to the urologist ever since Huggins, in 1939, first offered a new approach to the care of carcinoma of the prostate. More recently, Huggins and his associates proposed adrenalectomy for inoperable cancer, as well as hypophysectomy. Neither results have as yet been proven to be successful and further hormonal studies are now in progress. Of equal significance is that a great deal of experimental data seems to indicate that endocrine factors play a significant role in the pathogenesis of testicular tumors. Teratoma of the testis in the fowl can be produced by intratesticular injection of zinc or copper salts, but only when the animal's hormones are active in the Spring or when stimulated by injected pituitary hormones.

The role of hormonal influence appears apparent when one realizes that the incidence range of testicular cancer is basically from puberty to the fifth decade of life. It is rare after the sixth decade of life and extremely rare in childhood. It is most prevalent during the period of greatest sexual activity, namely between the thirty-fifth to the thirty-ninth year of life. It has been suggested that tumors with toti-potential cells (as in chorioepethelioma of the testes) are capable of secreting estrogens in addition to other hormonal substances.

Since the epochal discovery of chorionic gonadotropin by Ascheim and Zondek, subsequent investigations demonstrated that gonadotropic activity was present in the urine of young and old men as well as in menstruating and post-menopausal women. It is now more than a quarter of a century that sufficient data has been accumulated to indicate that the gonadotropic activity of the urine is of pituitary origin. Indeed, with the introduction of hypophysectomy as a palliative measure for cancer, direct evidence has been accumulated to show that the gonadotropic material of urine is derived from the pituitary gland.

Even though there is every reason to believe that testicular function may be influenced by, and in turn may influence, the behavior of other endocrine glands, all are agreed that testicular function is directly controlled by the anterior portion of the hypophysis (adenohypophysis). This singular gland stimulates the testis to secrete two hormones (a) follicle-stimulating hormone (F.S.H.) and (b) interstitial cell-stimulating hormone (I.C.S.H.) The F.S.H. stimulates and controls the development of the germinal epithelium at puberty and enables normal spermatogenesis to continue during adult life. When deficient or absent, spermatogenesis rarely goes beyond the stage of primary spermatocytes. The ICSH stimulates the cells of Leydig to produce testosterone. When this hormone is deficient or absent, secondary sexual characteristics do not develop and the external genitalia reveal the clinical picture of hypogonadism.

Of singular interest is that although spermatogenesis and the secretions of androgens occur somewhat independently of one another, it is now known that androgen secretion is necessary for normal spermatogenesis. Unfortunately elaborate studies in this direction are difficult for it is almost impossible to study spermatogenesis in the absence of normal Leydig cell function.

The sex of an individual is the result of two distinct processes, i.e., sex determination and sex differentiation. Sex determination is a genetic phenomenon and results in the sex genotype of the embryo. Sex differentiation is not a determination but is the course of events which occur during embryonic development, with an elaboration of homologous organs, accompanied by degeneration of heterologous counterparts, some of which may persist in the adult as vestigial remnants. In brief, sex differentiation refers to the changes which occur to the embryonic gonad, genital ducts and external genitalia. Genetic differentiation is the trial between the male and female elements in the potential bisexual embryonic gonad.

Anatomical anomalies as a result of endocrine disturbance may occur in infancy, at puberty or during adult life. Such disturbances are a serious challenge to the clinician, for faulty assignment of sex can lead to an unhappy socio-sexual adaptation. Fortunately, accurate sex typing is no longer dependent upon the obstetrician's decision, but is now more accurately determined by means of chromatin sex determination. When this is inadequate, laparotomy is justifiable and preferably at an early age (3-5 years).

It is known that in most species, the sex chromosomes contain conspicuous masses of heterochromatin. In a few species of insects, the heterochromatin persists in the intermitotic nucleus as a chromatin mass or masses. These masses are sufficiently characteristic to distinguish the nuclei of male from those of female insects. Barr and Bertram demonstrated this difference in the nerve cells of the hypoglossal nucleus of the cat. This gave rise to one of the most unusual and revealing techniques, based upon sex differences, in nucleus morphology of various cells. This method of nuclear sexing has been of tremendous value in the diagnosis of certain abnormalities. The most recent advance in this field of endocrinology has been the clarification of the trisonic syndromes only recently evaluated in medical literature.

The adreno-genital syndrome due to congenital adreno-cortical hyperplasia is another example of an inborn error of metabolism in man which now receives closer scrutiny and better understanding as to etiology and therapy. Since the introduction of the Zimmerman technique, it is now possible to accurately measure urinary 17-ketosteroids of adrenal origin, found to be elevated in these cases. With the administration of cortisones, it is possible to suppress the urinary 17-ketosteroid level and to clinically bring about remission of the disease. This is in contradiction to adrenal carcinoma with high levels of urinary 17-ketosteroids which cannot be suppressed by the administration of cortisone. Surgery of the adrenals is now possible only because of potent extracts now available for use as substitution therapy. This is important, for in many cases, surgical intervention, now feasible, is the only means of establishing the correct diagnosis.

Assays for urinary steroids are now recognized as indispensable to the diagnosis of adrenal and testicular disease. Values as to urinary steroids found in normal children, during the pre-puberal and post-puberal stage, and in adults are of great aid in differential diagnosis. This is in conjunction with x-ray (excretory pyelography, laminagraphy, or presacral air insufflation) has eliminated many questionable cases prior to surgical exploration.

Chapter 2

EMBRYONIC GONADAL DIFFERENTIATION

SOMATIC SEX DIFFERENTIATION, a term used to describe the development of the genital ducts and lower genital tract, is now universally accepted as a hormonal process. In this process the fetal testis plays an important role. Early[1,2,3] embryological experiments revealed that removal of the fetal ovary did not hinder differentiation of a female genital system, but that absence of the fetal testis and its *morphogenic hormone,* during an early critical uterine period prevented the differentiation of Wolffian derivatives and resulted in the development of the Müllerian ducts, urogenital sinus and female external genitalia. Thus it has been postulated that partial fetal insufficiency during the crucial phase of embryonic sex differentiation may lead to different phases and degrees of ambi-sexual development. In addition to the degree of testicular insufficiency, variations in time of removal, duration, and laterality of the deficiency of the *testicular morphogenetic hormone* determines the extent of the anomaly. As yet no clue has been detected as to the nature of this *morphogenetic hormone* of the testicle and until modern biochemical techniques can be applied to its structure, our knowledge of the mechanism of human sex differentiation will remain limited.*

---

*The theory stated above finds confirmation in the work of Jost[1] who carried out *in utero,* castration of rabbit embryos, in which the differentiation of the reproductive duct begins by 19-20 days of age, and is complete, to all intents and purposes, 2-3 days before birth. Jost showed that in males orchidectomized at 23-24 days of uterine development and killed at the 28 day, sexual differentiation had proceeded normally. If, on the other hand, the castration took place at an earlier stage, at the beginning of sexual differentiation, no male characteristics whatever developed. The Wolffian ducts disappeared entirely, while the prostate gland failed to develop and the external sexual organs were of a female type. The Müllerian ducts differentiated into the Müllerian vagina (an organ well developed in rabbits) the uterine horns, and sometimes the oviducts, but the size of these organs was less than in the normal female.

Jost[2,3] subsequently showed that the results of orchidectomy are associated with a defect in the humoral mechanism, and not with trauma or any unspecified influences what-

The first sexual primordium to appear is the gonadal anlage. It contains all structures essential for differentiation into either an ovary or a testis. This bipotential gonad[4,5,6] is composed of two somatic, unipotential primordia—a cortical element which is capable of developing only as an ovary, and a medullary element capable of becoming a testis. If the gonad is a testis, obviously the individual develops as a male; if an ovary, the individual is a female. If both testis and ovary are present, the individual is an hermaphrodite. This phase of development is referred to as the gonadal sex phase since the germ cells produced by a testis are spermatozoa and those produced by an ovary, ova. The sex of the gonad is actually imposed by the somatic part of the gland and not by the germinal cells.

Grumbach[7] points out that the concept of corticomedullary interaction or balance, with its mutually antagonistic physiologic relationship between the cortex and the medulla, has been well established in lower animals. If accepted, this concept has important implications as to the mechanism of reversal or inversion of gonadal development in man. To quote Grumbach,[7] "It affords an explanation of the occurrence of chromatin-positive persons with testes which may contain spermatozoa, of chromatin-negative persons with ovaries containing ovocytes and of either chromatin-negative or chromatin-positive persons with both ovarian and testicular tissue. Although the competitive relationship between cortex and medulla is gene controlled and the outcome normally is determined by genetic sex, a variety of experimental procedures can alter the balance between the cortex and the medulla contrary to genetic sex through inhibition of the dominant element."

---

soever, insofar as unilateral orchidectomy of the embryo of a male of 19-23 days did not in the least disturb the course of normal sexual differentiation. But in certain cases, the effect of the one remaining testicle after unilateral castration showed itself to be slightly weaker on the opposite testicleless side. From this, one could conclude that the determinant action of the fetal testis was local and not pervasive, as one would expect it to be, if it were the result of a hormonal influence. However, although there are many advocates of a gonadal endocrine influence operative during fetal life and although many of the intersex abnormalities are attributed to such influences, few of these hypotheses have been proven.

The first sexual anlage is identical regardless of the genetic sex of the embryo. It comes off the genital ridge from which the sex glands differentiate.[4] This undifferentiated gonad has two major somatic components, the cortex and the medulla, in addition to the germ cells. The medulla is concerned with testicular differentiation whereas the cortex influences ovarian differentiation. The medullary sex cords become evident in the embryo with a crown-rump length of 14-16 mm. These cells acquire a definite construction and become the seminiferous tubules of the testes. While this occurs the cortex (in the male) slowly degenerates.

In the female the cortex is the influencing factor, and as differentiation takes place the process is slower than when the indifferent gland changes to a testis. In ovarian development the cortex persists and actually increases in size. Somatic cells are found in the cortical cords, and there later becomes the granulosa cells, and germ cells, which later become the ovocytes.

Thus anlagen for the genital organs of both sexes exist in the early embryo and sexual differentiation occurs as a result of an orderly elaboration of homologous organs, together with degeneration of heterologous counterparts, some of which remain in the adult as vestigial remnants.[8]

After the sex glands are differentiated the genital tract undergoes a complete anatomical differentiation. "If we consider a young embryo at the time when sex differentiation of the gonad begins," states Jost,[1] "the urogenital system comprises the following parts. In the abdominal cavity, the mesonephros is the functioning kidney; the pronephros is represented only by more or less remains and the metanephros or definitive kidney is just differentiating. The mesonephric urinary duct, which we shall now call *Wolffian duct,* opens at its posterior end into a specialized part of the primitive *cloaca, the uro-genital sinus.* The primative urogenital ostium is separated from the rectum by the urorectal septum and is prolonged by a 'urethral groove' along the under surface of the genital tubule." As pointed out by Jost and others[1,2,3,4] it is at this time that a second pair of ducts, namely the Müllerian ducts, are developing on the anterior and external margin of the mesonephros. The fetus now has a double assortment of ducts, a primitive urogenital sinus and a genital tubercle, but embryologically is sexually undifferentiated as to a definite functioning genital tract.

As soon as sexual differentiation begins, specific parts retrogress and other parts become incorporated into the genital system. For example, in the female, the Wolffian ducts do not become sexual structures but retrogress along with the mesonephros. Some tubules of the mesonephros near the ovary, persist as the epoophoron. The Müllerian ducts do not regress. They persist as tubes and uterus. From the urogenital sinus (in the female) contributions are made to the female urethra and vagina.

This "somatic sexual differentiation" is quite different in the male. For example, the mesonephric or Wolffian ducts do not regress but become part of the sexual system. The vas deferentia comes from the free part of the Wolffian ducts and from its opposite and produces diverticula which become the seminal vesicles. Differing from the female, in the male the Müllerian ducts disappear rather quickly. From the urogenital sinus, contributions are made to form the prostate and male urethra.

The external genitalia similarly goes through a phase of sexual differentiation followed by permanent sexual differentiation. Early in fetal life the external genitalia consist essentially of (a) a genital tubercle or phallus; (b) a urethral groove, which is limited by two urethral folds; and (c) the genital swellings on either side of the phallus.

When the foetus reaches two months, sex differentiation is first detectable. In the male, fusion of the urethral folds occurs, first in the pelvic region, ultimately bringing the urogenital ostium onto the phallus, toward the glans penis. This produces a perineal raphe, which extends from the urogenital ostium to the anus. At this phase the scrotal swelling is more perineal and away from the base of the phallus. As the foetus grows larger (70 mm.) the preputial folds and the corpora cavernosa become differentiated and by the fourth month the external genitalia are clearly developed. However, the testes remain in the abdomen and do not descend into the scrotum until early in the seventh month.

Sex differentiation in the female progresses by the urethral groove remaining open and developing as the vulva. In contrast to the male, the urethral folds do not fuse, but instead form the labia minora. The genital (labial) folds (in the male scrotal swellings) become elongated and flank the base of the clitoris (labia majora). All of these features are clearly distinguishable as female characteristics when the foetus is ninety days.

Despite the great strides made in embryological research the basic cause of sexual abnormalities in the human still remains unsolved. The exact definition of the abnormality is difficult and one can only agree with Jost[1] when he says, "It finally appears that the development of the somatic sexual organs may present defects resulting in either malformations of their primordia or, more frequently, from endocrine impairments occurring at definite stages of intrauterine life." *When one considers the complex embryological development of the testicle and ovary it is amazing that more complex mal-developments do not occur and that actual sexual anomalies are not more prevalent.*

The role of the Müllerian ducts in the female and the Wolffian ducts in the male play an important role in the differentiation and development of the sex glands. The degree of differentiation or suppression of the Müllerian and Wolffian ducts depends upon the presence or absence of functioning fetal testes during the early stages of fetal development. It is believed that differentiation of the external genitals may be altered by early function of the fetal testes, congenital adrenal hyperplasia of the fetus, hyperandrogenic conditions in the mother, or by intrinsic embryological defects.

Wiesner[7] has postulated the so-called "monohormonic" theory of morphological differentiation which has supplanted the so-called "dihormonic" theory based on the classic study of Lillie[18] on the bovine free-martin.* The "monohormonic" theory is: The presence or absence of the fetal testes is of primary significance in normal sex differentiation, and that, if the so-called fetal testes are absent or do not function during the early embryonic stages, Müllerian ducts develop and Wolffian ducts are suppressed with differentiation of the external genitalia in a gynecoid fashion.

---

*The interested reader is strongly recommended to read Moore's *Lecture on Embryonic Sex Hormones and Sexual Differentiation.*[24]

Hamblen[10] cites that simulant females with gonadal aplasia or hypoplasia and with chromatin-negative patterns, apparently providing clinical confirmation of Jost's data, points out that Grumbach and associates suggests that the preponderance of chromatin-negative individuals in this syndrome indicates that the fetal testes, "particularly its germinal elements, may be more susceptible to damage from some unknown cause in early uterine life than the fetal ovary."

"The findings of anorchia," continues Hamblen,[10] "upon careful surgical exploration of morphologically normal males who were presumed to be cryptorchid would seem to negate the clinical application of the data of Jost. However, a logical assumption is that testes were present during the critical period of these individual's sexual differentiation and that they were subsequently degenerated, probably during their descent through the inguinal canals." In 1956, Amelar[12] reported a case of anorchism without eunuchism. This case is of singular importance for it is the only one in the literature of proven anorchism in which a young male adult (19) presents psychosexual development along masculine lines, with normal male sexual urges and ability to have ejaculations. This is explained on a basis of the finding of extra-testicular (Leydig) cells scattered along the Wolffian duct structures in the inguinal canals, and it is quite logical to assume these cells probably represent the remnants of degenerated testes. All other cases[13, 14] of anorchism reported in the literature reveal: (1) absence of sex desire, (2) absence of erections, (3) absence of emissions, (4) feminine voice, (5) scanty or absent facial or pubic hair, (6) small penis, (7) small empty scrotum; and (8) empty inguinal canals.

Overzier[15] has described a theory which in a way supplements Jost's[1, 2, 3] concept of the role of the fetal testes in sexual differentiation. It is as follows: "The first anlage of the gonads stimulate the first anlage of the Wolffian and Müllerian ducts, probably even at a time before the anatomical structure can be recognized (Initial Induction). Constructions of the male or female duct system follows as a result of Permanent Induction by the further developing gonads. If Permanent Induction is lacking, as after experimental castration in early foetal life or as in Turner's syndrome, whether the individual is genetically male or genetically female, the ducts develop in the female direction from the stimulus of the Initial Induction. Yet if Initial Induction is also lacking, as in true agonadism, where there is no gonadal anlage, the Wolffian and Müllerian ducts persist as co-existing, underdeveloped structures." This theory is supported by experimental and clinical evidence including the author's personal observation of two genetically male siblings with true agonadism—first case of this kind in the international literature.

The experiments of Stockard[16] are of interest for they show the role of blighting. Stockard and his workers have demonstrated that if the egg of the marine minnow Fundulus is cooled at a certain stage of development a perfect twin will be developed, but if cooled at a later time, will form instead an imperfect embryo. These workers have been able to demonstrate that with the use of temperature, chemicals, anoxia and other agents, fusions, duplications, local overgrowths and suppressions of the several organ systems have been produced.

The human fetus similarly can be affected by changes in maternal metabolism or by variations in the placental circulation. Thus, as emphasized by Hinman,[17] if these blighting influences occur at the exact moment of ascent of the female urethral plate, the phallic portion may close over and form an anomalous penile urethra. Hinman states, "conceivably, any genital anomaly is possible. Actually, only a few major patterns appear: (1) true hermaphroditism, with development of male and female gonads; (2) intersexuality of the vaginal urethral type, with phallic urethra; and (3) extreme anomalous development approaching monster formation, with gross genital and other malformation."

The unexpected occurrence of partial masculinization of the female fetus, associated with treatment of pregnant women with androgens, has provided a unique opportunity to study the hormonal influence on the female fetus in the human. Wilkins[19] *et al.*, have reported the occurrence of partial masculinization of the external genitalia in female infants whose mothers were given oral 17-ethynlytestosterone or parenteral progesterone. Grumbach[20, 21] and Ducharme studied eighteen cases of partial masculinization of the female fetus associated with oral progestin therapy, and following their original investigation[20] do not recommend the use of oral progestins that exhibit androgenic activity in the female fetus. In this respect Jones and Wilkins[22] recommend that the use of progestogen should be reserved only for those cases where a progestogenic deficiency can be shown to exist, and emphasize that the defect is not serious, and can be easily corrected, but that awareness of the problem is important.

SUMMARY

(1) The sex of an individual is the result of two distinct processes, i.e., sex determination and sex differentiation.

(2) Sex determination is the sex genotype of the embryo.

(3) Sex differentiation is not a determination but is the course of events which occur during embryonic development, with an elaboration of homologous organs, accompanied by degeneration of heterologous counterparts, some of which may persist in the adult as vestigial remnants.

(4) Sex differentiation refers to the changes which occur to the embryonic gonad, genital ducts and external genitalia.

(5) Sex differentiation is the trial between male and female elements in the potential bisexual embryonic gonad.

(6) Gonadal dysgenesis should be suspected whenever there is any doubt concerning the external genitalia of an infant or young child.

(7) The diagnosis usually is confirmed by the finding of male nuclear chromatin pattern in the buccal and vaginal cells of infants with normal-appearing female external genitalia.[23] Even if the pattern is positive, consideration of the diagnosis should be continued, especially if other features are demonstrable.

(8) A newborn infant with ambiguous external genitalia must be suspected of having female hermaphroditism (nonvirilizing). When the nuclear chromatin test is positive, one must consider in the differential diagnosis: (1) the adrenogenital syndrome (see subsequent chapters), (2) true hermaphroditism, and (3) nonvirilizing female hermaphroditism. Adrenal hyperplasia can be ruled out if there is a normal excretion of urinary 17-ketosteroids.

True hermaphroditism can only be eliminated by laparotomy. With a history of maternal progestogen therapy, laparotomy is not indicated.

(9) Where the hermaphroditism is the result of steroid therapy (maternal) progressive virilization does not occur. "Although no patient with iatrogenic masculinized external genitalia has yet reached puberty, there is no reason to believe any abnormality in menstruation will ensue. For these reasons the rearing should be feminine."[22]

REFERENCES

1. Jost, A.: Recherches sur la differenciation sexuelle de l'embryon de lapin. III Role des gonades foetales dans la differenciation sexuelle somatique. *Arch. Anat. Micr. et Morphol. Expér., 36:* 271, 1947.
2. Jost, A.: Problems of fetal endocrinology: the gonadal and hypophyseal hormones. *Recent Progr. Horm. Res., 8:* 379, 1953.
3. Jost, A.: Hormonal factors in the development of the fetus. Cold Spring Harbor Symp. *Quant. Biol., 19:* 167, 1954.
4. Arey, H. B.: *Developmental Anatomy.* W. B. Saunders, Philadelphia, 1948.
5. Gruenwald, P.: Development of Sex Cords in Gonads of Man and Mammals. *Am. J. Anat., 70:* 359, 1942.
6. Willier, B. H.: Embryonic Development of Sex. In *Sex and Internal Secretions,* The Williams and Wilkins Co., Baltimore, 1939.
7. Grumbach, M.: The Sex Chromatin Pattern and Human Sexual Anomalies. *Year Book of Endocrinology,* 1958-1959, p. 290-291.
8. Hall, P. F.: The Functions of the Endocrine Glands. Chapter 4, *The Testes.* W. B. Saunders Co., Philadelphia, 1959.
9. Wiesner, B. P.: The post natal development of the genital organs in the albino rat, with a discussion of a new theory of sexual differentiation. *J. Obst. & Gynec. Brit. Emp., 41:* 867-929, *42:* 8-78, 1934, 1935.
10. Hamblen, E. C.: The assignment of sex to an individual: Some enigmas and some practical clinical criteria. *Am. J. of Obs. and Gynecol.,* Vol. *74,* No. 6, 1228-1244, Dec., 1957.
11. Grumbach, M. M., and Ducharme, J. R.: Effects of androgens on fetal sexual development: Androgen-induced Female Pseudohermaphroditism, *J. Clin. Endocrinol., 19:* 1369-1380, Nov., 1950.
12. Amelar, R. D.: Anorchism without eunuchism. *J. Urol., 76:* No. 2, p. 174, 1956.
13. Counseller, U. S., and Walker, M. S.: Congenital absence of testes. *Ann. Surg., 98:* 104-109, 1933.

14. Hepburn, R. H.: Anorchism. *J. Urol., 62:* 65, 1949.
15. Overzier, C.: Problems in Inter sexuality concerning the sexual ducts in true agonadism, gonadal dysgenesis and Turner's syndrome. *Symposium on Nuclear Sex.* Interscience Publishers, Inc. New York, 1958.
16. Stockard, C. R.: Developmental Rate and Structural Expression: An Experimental Study of Twins, "Double Monsters" and Single Deformities and the Interaction among Embryonic Organs during their Origin and Development. *Am. J. Anat., 28:* 115, 1921.
17. Hinman, Jr., F.: *Intersexuality.* The Pediatric Clinics of North America. Philadelphia, Saunders Co., Nov., 1957.
18. Lillie, F. R.: The free martin, a study of the action of sex hormones in the foetal life of cattle. *J. Exper. Zool., 23:* 371, 1917.
19. Wilkins, L., Jones, H. W., Jr., Holman, G. H., and Stempfel, R. S., Jr.: Masculinization of the female fetus associated with administration of oral and intramuscular progestins during gestation; non-adrenal female pseudohermaphroditism. *J. Clin. Endocrinol., 18:* 559, 1958.
20. Grumbach, M. M., Ducharme, J. R., and Moloshok, R. E.: On the fetal masculinizing action of certain oral progestins. *J. Clin. Endocrinol., 19:* 1369, 1959.
21. Grumbach, M. M., and Ducharme, J. R.: The effects of androgens on fetal sexual development, *J. Fertility and Sterility, 11:* 157, 1960.
22. Jones, H. W., and Wilkins, L.: The genital anomaly associated with prenatal exposure to progestogens. *J. Fertility and Sterility, 11:* 148, 1960.
23. Grumbach, M. M., and Barr, M. L.: Cytological tests of chromosomal sex in relation to sexual anomalies in man. *Rec. Prog. in Hormone Research, 14:* 255, 1958.
24. Moore, C. R.: *Embryonic Sex Hormones and Sexual Differentiation.* Thomas, Springfield, 1947.

Chapter 3

HORMONAL INFLUENCES IN GONADAL DIFFERENTIATION AND GROWTH

THE DEVELOPMENT of a somatic sexual organ, as the testicle, may be subject to defects which may be the result of (1) some anatomical congenital malformation or (2) some endocrine influence either during intra-uterine life or during the post natal phase of life. The latter may occur because of faulty hormonal synthesis or a change in the responsiveness of the tissue.

The glands of internal secretion are of great significance, particularly in childhood where they have three major functions: (1) to stimulate growth; (2) to influence metabolic activities; and (3) to regulate physical changes leading to adolescence. Thus, it is said that development in normal youth is essentially a problem of normal activity of the pituitary gland and the ability of the target glands to respond to its stimulations. The male gonads and female gonads are vital target glands highly susceptible to stimulation from the anterior pituitary gland, which elaborates substances known as gonadotropins. These substances have been identified and assayed in human male pituitary glands.[1]

In the following discussion, emphasis will be placed upon the nature of the gonadotropins in man and the accepted factors which influence their secretion. These hormones are controlled both from above and below, i.e., from suprasellar centers in the brain and gonadal secretions.

Normal gonadal activity is dependent upon anterior pituitary gonadotropic hormone stimulation. The male has two gonadotropins: (1) the follicle stimulating hormone (FSH) which induces spermatic tubule development and spermatogenesis; and (2) the interstitial cell-stimulating hormone (ICSH) which stimulates the testicular interstitial cells to develop and initiate androgen (Leydig cells) production by the testis. Here it is of interest to note that a hormone similar to ICSH in action has been extracted from human urine during pregnancy. Since its derivation has been traced to the placental chorion, it is called "Chorionic gonadotropic" and because of its resemblance to pituitary ICSH it has been called the "anterior-pituitary-like" hormone. At times chorionic gonadotropin is substituted for ICSH and used therapeutically.

Fetal testicular activity is closely associated with exposure to both endogenous and exogenous gonadotropic hormones. *Thus,* from the moment of its differentiation, the fetal testis is exposed to a significant quantity of chorionic gonadotropin. Although of trophoblastic origin, Segal and Nelson,[2] believe this hormone should be considered as an external stimulus to the fetus. The hormone is believed to enter the fetal septum across the wall of the chorionic vesicle by seepage into the fetal fluids, rather than through the umbilical circulation. Bruner[3] believes that the amount of chorionic gonadotropin in the fetal body as early as 11 weeks of age is physiologically significant, and this assumption is supported by the morphologic stimulation of the interstitium of the fetal testis during late pregnancy and its post-partum regression. At about the eighth month, the Leydig cells show hypertrophy and secretory activity, which many believe actually contributes to the descent of the testes into the scrotum at this time. Confirmation of such activity is further evidenced by the fact that shortly (5 days) after the fetus leaves its uterine environment the Leydig cells regress, so that they are not again identifiable until the onset of puberty.

The FSH which induces spermatic tubule development and spermatogenesis is not secreted by the anterior pituitary* during

---

*The anterior pituitary gland exerts a marked influence upon the testicle as well as other endocrine structures, and for this reason is usually regarded as the *master gland.* It is located within the sella turcica of the sphenoid bone, surrounded by the dura mater. It is attached to the floor of the third ventricle by a thin stalk, where it lies in close proximity to the optic chiasma. The British usually refer to the anterior pituitary gland as the adenohypophysis and the term neurohypophysis is applied to the posterior portion of the pituitary gland.

the preadolescent period. During this period the tubules are immature and quiescent. However, during adolescence the *Pituitary* secretes increased amounts of FSH as demonstrated by the finding of increased amounts in the urine. When the male reaches adolescence, disturbances of the testicular tubules brings about compensatory alteration in FSH production. Further, if the individual is castrated or has extensive damage to the spermatic tubules, the urinary gonadotropins become markedly increased.* FSH production by the pituitary can be inhibited by the administration of estrogen, an action which has not yet been satisfactorily explained. At puberty FSH excretion in the urine approaches the adult level of about 60 mouse units in 24 hours.

Nathanson[4] *et al.*, in a study of normal excretion of sex hormones in childhood, have summarized the following interesting data: (1) From 3-7 years of age both boys and girls excrete a small and constant amount of estrogens and 17-ketosteroids in the urine with little difference between the sexes; (2) from 7-11 years of age more 17-ketosteroids found in the urine of boys than girls; (3) about 1½ years before the menarche, estrogen excretion becomes cyclic in girls, and the intensity of these cycles gradually increases; (4) in boys after 11 years of age with secondary characteristics there is an increase of 17-ketosteroids in the urine; and (5) at 11 years of age the FSH of the anterior pituitary gland is first detected in the urine of girls, but in boys it appears somewhere between the ages of 12 and 13 years.

There is some evidence that a second hormone of the testis is secreted under the influence of FSH. This hormone has been referred to as "X-hormone" and "inhibin." Some believe that estrogen is secreted by the testis and that this may be the second hormone. Confirmation of this theory is still awaited, but there is evidence to believe that estrogen is present in the testis of the bull[12] and the stallion[13] and estradiol[14] has been isolated from human testes.

*In Klinefelter's syndrome, the tubules are often completely hyalinized. In spite of this there is clinical evidence of normal levels of circulating androgens and normal urinary 17-ketosteroid excretion. However the urinary gonadotropins are found at high levels.[11]

The need of the testicle being in the scrotum for maturation of the testicular tubules and ultimate spermatogenesis becomes apparent when it is realized that sterility, testicular atrophy, torsion, hernia and testicular tumors are more prone in the undescended testicle. This will be discussed later, but it would not be amiss to point out here that in cryptorchidism the tubules remain immature in spite of the fact the androgen may be secreted normally and virilization occurs. Thus, even though there is atrophy and degeneration of the tubular lining, which may also occur in x-radiation, mumps orchitis and Klinefelter's syndrome, the interstitial cells (Leydig) are unimpaired and continue to function sufficiently to sustain secondary sexual development although spermatogenesis is impaired if not completely destroyed. The seminiferous tubules are extremely sensitive to agents of various kinds, whereas the cells of Sertoli and the Leydig cells (interstitial cells) are relatively resistant to such agents.

The fate of the castrated male has been known to mankind for many hundreds of years. Loss of the testes (prior to puberty) produces an alteration in the pitch of the voice and a loss of sexual drive. It makes the skin texture smooth and without hair. Of course, such an individual is unable to procreate. Berthold[5] in 1849, was the first to demonstrate that the testis secretes a hormone, when he succeeded in preventing postcastration atrophy of the cock's comb by implanting the excised testis in a location where it could re-establish a new circulation.

Under normal circumstances the adolescent male undergoes certain endocrinologic changes which alter his facial appearance, voice, breasts and configuration of body as well as distribution of hair. The penis becomes larger both in length and diameter and the testes increase in size. The reader must recall that in perfectly normal adolescent males the larynx and facial hair follicles may not respond to circulating hormones. Such males have a high-pitched, puerile voice and are beardless but they are thoroughly masculine and able to reproduce. The adolescent age may vary and no definite age can be given for these changes to occur other than to suggest that most boys begin to mature between the ages of 12 and 16 years.

These changes are accelerated at the time of puberty; but are dependent upon certain hormonal cycles and balances. Thus, the male sex hormone produced by the interstitial cells of Leydig, is more significant in the endocrine physiology of the male. Even though androgenic hormones are secreted by the cortex of the adrenal, it is the testicular secretion which is important. This hormone in turn is dependent upon adequate stimulation from the pituitary gonadotropic hormone (ICSH).

SEXUAL RETARDATION

Obviously when a young boy exhibits signs of delayed sexual and somatic development a great deal of anxiety on the part of the parents is aroused. For example, the male child of 13 or 14 who does not begin to show signs outlined above, and who continues to show an absence of such signs for a period of about two years is a typical example of adolescent retardation. As a rule the history will reveal that the father, uncle or other member of the family exhibited the same type of delayed adolescence. This is not of a permanent nature for ultimately such individuals mature quite normally. It is only an expression of a delay in the pituitary-gonadal-adrenal axis. Indeed many of these patients make rapid strides in growth and sexual maturity once adolescence is begun.

The problem is to be able to distinguish between the young male with delayed adolescence and the young male who will remain permanently immature sexually and physically because of hormonal deficiency. Here a careful examination of the testes with progressive enlargement, even though slow, and the finding of urinary 17-ketosteroids comparable to level found in normal adolescence as well as a normal output of FSH assures the physician that it is retardation, rather than pituitary infantilism or other hormonal deficiency.[6, 7]

"The mechanism which is responsible for the initiation of puberty is poorly understood," states Wilkins.[8] "Apparently at this time neural or neurohumoral stimuli from the hypothalamus cause the secretion of gonadotropin hormones by the anterior pituitary. Some workers believe that during immaturity there is an inhibition of this mechanism. It is probable that a certain degree of physiologic maturation of the nervous system must be maintained before the infantile inhibition is released or the hypothalamic-pituitary mechanism becomes active. The developmental changes of the central nervous system might be likened to those responsible during infancy for motor performances, speech development and sphincter control."

Steckel[9] gives data about the average approximate age and sequence of appearance of sexual characteristics in the following manner: Ages 10 to 11, first growth of testes and penis; 13 to 14, rapid growth of testes and penis, subareolar node of nipples; 14 to 15, axillary hair, down on upper lip; 15 to 16, mature spermatozoa (average 15 years) (Range 11¼ to 17); 16 to 17, facial and body hair, acne; and at 21, arrest of skeletal growth.

The testicular or male hormone, produced by the interstitial cells of the testis, and quite independent of spermatogenesis, is essential for normal development of male characteristics. A disturbance in the adequate productions of androgens (secreted in the form of testosterone) results in an inability for maintenance of structure and functions of the male gonad.[10]

One would assume that if there is any doubt as to the status of androgenic function in a young male, confirmation would not be difficult. Unfortunately it is difficult because clinical findings alone are inadequate and also because of the wide range of normal among puberal boys and men. In addition, testicular and androgenic function unfortunately cannot be determined with quantitative precision, for approximately two-thirds of the androgenic substances in the urine probably have their origin in the adrenal cortex.

Testicular biopsy offers a method of truly evaluating the male gonad. This will be discussed more fully in a later section. It is a valuable and accurate clinical method of determining the exact status of the male gonad and indirectly evaluating the hormonal status of the young male.

SUMMARY

(1) Although it is accepted that testicular function can be influenced by other endocrine glands, whose behavior it may also

influence, it is fair to assume that testicular function is directly influenced by the anterior pituitary gland.

(2) The anterior pituitary can stimulate the testicular secretion of two important hormones; (a) follicle-stimulating hormone (FSH); (b) interstitial cell-stimulating hormone (ICSH).

(3) FSH stimulates the development of the germinal epithelium at puberty and allows for normal spermatogenesis during adult life.

(4) ICSH, stimulates the cells of Leydig to produce testosterone which enables secondary sexual characteristics to develop as well as allows for normal genital development.

(5) Spermatogenesis and the secretion of androgens occur independently.

(6) It is believed by some that the seminiferous tubules may produce hormones, and thus add an additional function to the testicular tubule besides sperm production.

REFERENCES

1. Witschi, E., and Riley, G. M.: Quantitative studies on hormones of human pituitaries, *Endocrin., 26,* 565, 1940.
2. Segal, S. J., and Nelson, W. O.: *Initiation and Maintenance of Testicular Function.* Conference on Recent Progress in the Endocrinology of Reproduction. Edited by Lloyd, C. W. Academic Press, Inc. New York and London, 1959.
3. Bruner, J. A.: Distribution of chorionic gonadotropin in mother and fetus at various stages of pregnancy. *J. Clin. Endocrinol., 11:* 360-374, 1951.
4. Nathanson, I. T., Towne, L. E., and Aub, J. C.: Normal excretion of sex hormones in children. *Endocrin., 28:* 851, 1941.
5. Berthold, A. A.: Transplantation der Hoden. *Arch. f. Anat., Physiol. u. Wissensch. Med.,* pp. 426, 1849.
6. Williams, R. H.: *Textbook of Endocrinology.* Philadelphia, W. B. Saunders Co., 1955.
7. Soffer: *Diseases of the Endocrine Glands.* 2nd Edition. Lea and Febiger, 1959.
8. Wilkins, L.: *The Diagnosis and Treatment of Endocrine Disorders in Childhood and Adolescence,* 2nd Ed. Thomas, Springfield, 1957.
9. Steckel: Reference from Wilkins, L.: *Diagnosis in Childhood and Adolescence,* 2nd Ed. Thomas, Springfield, 1957.
10. Hall, P. F.: The Functions of the Endocrine Glands. Chapter 4, p. 75-96. *The Testes.* W. B. Saunders, Co., Philadelphia, 1959.

11. McCullagh, P. E., and Schaffenburg, A. C.: The role of the seminiferous tubules in the production of hormones. *Ann. of the New York Acad. of Sc., 55:* 674, 1952.
12. Dorfman, R. I., Gallagher, F. T., and Koch, C. F.: Nature of estrogenic substance in human male urine and bull testes. *Endocrinol., 19:* 33, 1935.
13. Beall, D.: Isolation of alpha-estradiol and estrone from horse testes. *Biochem. J., 34:* 1293, 1940.
14. Goldzieher, J. W., and Roberts, S. I.: Identification of steroids in human testes. Assoc. Study Internal Secretions, 33rd meeting, Atlantic City, N. J., 1951.

Chapter 4

TESTICULAR DEVELOPMENTAL HISTOLOGY

THE MICROSCOPIC appearance of the testicle is of great clinical significance.* Prior to the advent of *testicular biopsies*, knowledge of the true histological development of the testicle was meagre and inadequate.** The histologic picture of the infantile testicle, the prepuberal and postpuberal testicle can now be evaluated and classified as to inadequate or adequate testicular development.[2,3,4,5,6] In this section special emphasis will be given to the histologic appearance of the testis from birth through adolescence.

Testicular biopsy[3,4] originally devised as a method of diagnosis, in cases where no sperm were found or where the number of sperm were reduced to only an occasional cell per high power microscopic field, is now also utilized in conjunction with nuclear staining for positive identification of indicated sex assignment and better understanding of testicular endocrinopathies. This is of significant value in Klinefelter's[7] syndrome, as well as in other endocrine disturbances involving the male gonad. Testicular biopsy is a helpful guide if there is doubt about a person's sex, and is of distinct aid to differential diagnosis of intersex and hypogonadism.

TECHNIQUE FOR TESTICULAR BIOPSY

Testicular biopsy is a simple procedure which can be performed in the office, out-patient department, or, as performed by the author, in the operating room. Local or pentothal anesthesia is most

*The growth of our knowledge of the histophysiology of the testis has been closely tied to the development of new methods for the study of its structure. Improvements in methods of fixation and microtomy have now made it possible to bring the high resolving power of the electron microscope to bear upon the remaining problems in the finer structure of the testis.[1]

**The reader interested in a comprehensive discussion of electron microscopy (ultra violet light microscopy and fluorescent anti-body method of microscopy) is referred to a recent symposium, "History of Microscopy—1490 to the Present."[22]

adequate. The author has frequently performed this innocuous procedure in the cystoscopy room after pan-endoscopic studies, utilizing a separate sterile table set up with lap drapes, towels, tincture merthiolate, scissors, hand forceps, small clamps, black silk and triple zero atraumatic sutures. No preparation is needed other than a soap and water scrub and application of tincture of merthiolate to the scrotal area.

The testis is grasped between the thumb and second and third fingers of the left hand. With gentle but firm tension the scrotal skin is placed on the stretch, forcing the testis to be immobilized immediately beneath the skin. With a small scalpel the skin and subcutaneous tissue is cut until the tunica albugenia is exposed. This is then incised for about 2 centimeters which then allows for escape of clear fluid (always encountered and sometimes resembling a true hydrocele). After incising thru the tunica albugenia for about one centimeter, the seminiferous tubules, yellow in color, are now seen to extrude through the wound.* With scissors a tubular mass about the size of a pinhead is trimmed off. This is immediately dropped into a fixative of 5% glacial acetic acid in Zenkers solution, with appropriate label of name of patient, hospital number and side of biopsy. If performed bilaterally, separate bottles should be used and the side identified. The left hand is now relaxed and the tubules drop back within the testis and the testis retracts within the skin.

Small bleeding points are ligated. As a rule no bleeding occurs and if present may be controlled with pressure or with an atraumatic tie. No sutures are placed in the testis and the skin is closed with one black silk suture. The author recommends a small dry sterile gauze and a properly fitted surgical suspensory. The same procedure is carried out on the opposite side. Sutures may be removed within 3-5 days and if triple zero absorbable sutures are used in the skin, they will be found to be absorbed within one week. If patient is ambulatory he is allowed to remain quite for one hour and is given codeine sulfate, half grain,

---

*Too often incomplete incision of the tunica albugenia will result in inadequate biopsy and no seminiferous tubules or extra-tubular cellular structures will be visualized.

and aspirin, ten grains. He is then allowed to go home but advised to restrain from any physical exertion for the remainder of the day.

In the child the technic for obtaining the biopsy is essentially the same as for testicular biopsy in the adult. However, it may at times prove a little more difficult to obtain a specimen in the child because the immature testicular tissue does not bulge (as in the adult). When the tunica is incised it is necessary to scoop the tissue out. Regardless of this change in technique the reaction to the operative trauma is no more than in the adult. This is important, and if stressed to the parents, permission for biopsy will be more than willingly obtained.

As pointed out by Simmons,[2] interpretation of the testicular biopsy is a relatively new subject. "In general," states Simmons,[2] "testicular biopsy is indicated in those patients who have complete azoospermia in the seminal fluid, on more than one examination; and in patients who have marked oligospermia who do not respond to simple therapeutic measures in a six months' period. It also has a distinct place in the differential diagnosis of various endocrine disorders, such as eunuchoidism with negative FSH, male climacteric complete aspermatogenesis, spermatogenic arrest, and allied conditions." The testicular biopsy is of great help in evaluating the effects of various endocrine therapies. In such cases the biopsy is taken before, during and after a course of hormone therapy. As a rule, if both gonads are of the same size testicular biopsy of one should represent the spermatogenic activity of both testes. Simmons[2] and others,[3,4,5,7] believe that bilateral testicular biopsy be performed, wherever possible, to establish the premise biostatistically. The procedure is a harmless one, and it is in my opinion, indicated, whenever there is any doubt as to the fertility of the male and his hormonal status. It should be performed bilaterally.[8,9]

The histologic appearance of the testis from ages 3½ weeks to 4 years (referred to as the static phase by Charney and Wolgin)[10] varies little and is so similar that this age span can be taken as a single group and described as follows: The seminiferous tubules are small, about 66 microns in diameter. Only slight tortuosity exists. The tubules are lined with small, undifferentiated ovoid or

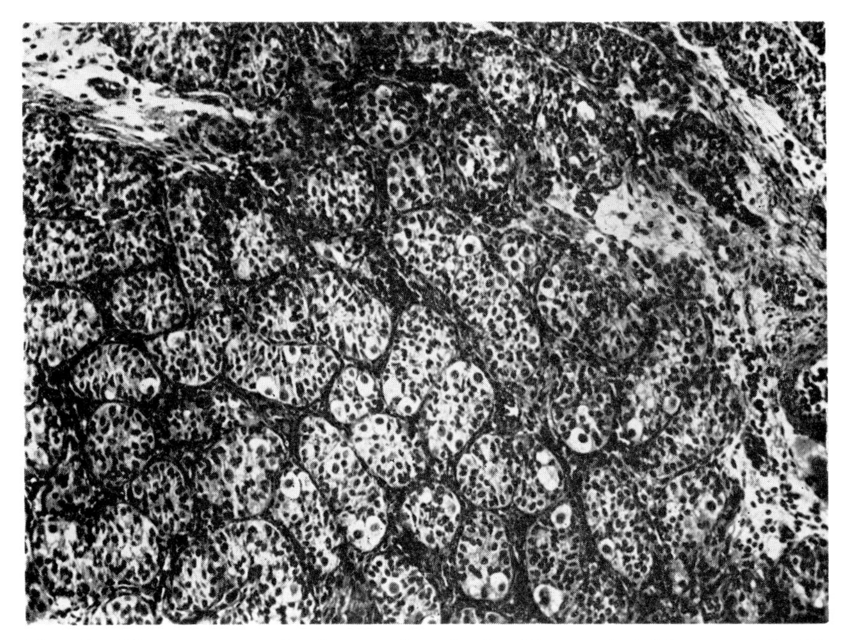

FIG. 1. Photomicrograph of normal testicular biopsy of child one week old. The seminiferous tubules are small, but have identifiable lumen formation with many small undifferentiated ovoid cells. No tortuosity exists and no Leydig cells are identified. Compare this section with Figures 2, 3, and 4.

cuboidal cells (later phase identified as spermatogonia). Lumen formation can be identified in approximately one-half of the tubules. No Leydig cells are identified. Leydig cells are seen in the new born infant probably due to maternal gonadotropin stimulation but rapidly disappear after birth.

In the next phase of growth, ages 5 to 9 the seminiferous tubules are still small but now show increasing tortuosity and have an average diameter of about 78 mm. The tubules are now lined in a more orderly fashion. A basement membrane can be identified. Spermatogonia and Sertoli cells are now identified but Leydig cells are not present.

With further development and maturation a marked change is now seen in the histological picture.[11,12,13] Spermatogonia and later primary spermatocytes are seen. At age 11 secondary spermatocytes are seen, and one year later numerous spermatids can

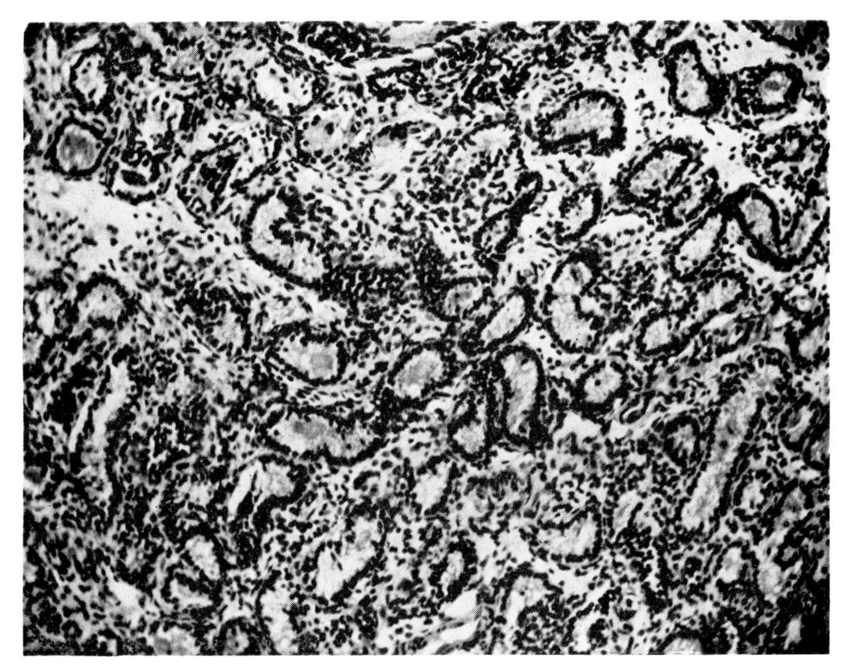

FIG. 2. Photomicrograph of testicular biopsy of child 3½ years of age. The seminiferous tubules are small with slight tortuosity and have definite lumen formation. The tubules are lined with small, undifferentiated ovoid or cuboidal cells. Leydig cells are not identified.

be identified. Of singular interest is that at approximately age 10, Leydig cells are first seen in the interstitial tissue. Thus it can be said that testis maturation begins at age 10 and progresses over a period of 2-4 years until completed.

From ages 11 to 15 the seminiferous tubules become larger in diameter, 100 to 150 microns (average adult tubule size 150 to 180 microns) and more tortuous.[11, 12, 13] Active spermatogenesis occurs up to and including the manufacture of a few spermatozoa. Leydig cells are abundantly found in the interstitial tissue. Since the age of puberty is a variable one, depending upon many inherent factors, racial and geographic influences, as well as hormonal status, it cannot be confined to one age. The progressive increase in an orderly fashion of the number of tubules, its size, cellular elements and active spermatogenesis is obvious. Of particular

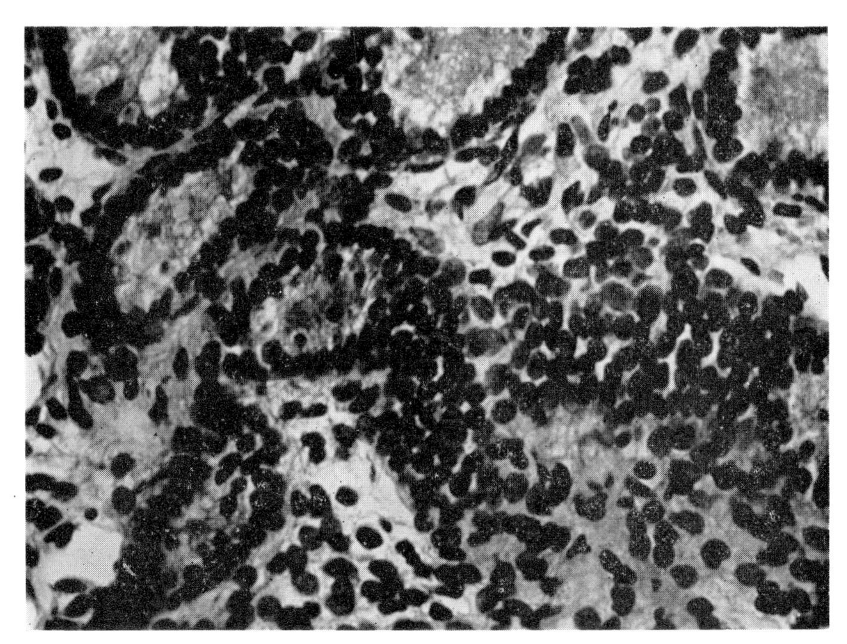

FIG. 3. Same as Figure 2 under high power. Incipient lumen formation is seen in more than half the tabules. No demonstrable Leydig cells.

endocrine significance is that the first appearance of true tubular development occurs at age 10. At this age, it is first possible to identify gonadotropins and 17-ketosteroids in an appreciable amount in the urine.

The first evidence of puberty in the testis is the formation of the tubular tunica propria.[8] In the absence of male sex hormone activity, this structure never forms, as is the case in hypergonadotropic eunuchoids even in the 4th and 5th decades of life. When one sees evidence of the tunica propria being deposited in young boys, one can predict rather confidently that within the next year or so other evidences of puberty will be manifested. Actually the tunica propria develops before initiation of spermatogenesis.

Spermatogenesis is accomplished step by step during puberty. It is first demonstrated by increasing numbers of spermatogonia which line the basement membrane. Subsequently primary and then secondary spermatocytes, spermatids, and sperm are developed. At about this time, recognizable Leydig cells develop from the mesenchymal cells in great numbers. Actually more are seen at this age than in the adult testis. Full maturation with adult characteristics of the interstitial tissue usually occurs at about 17 years of age.

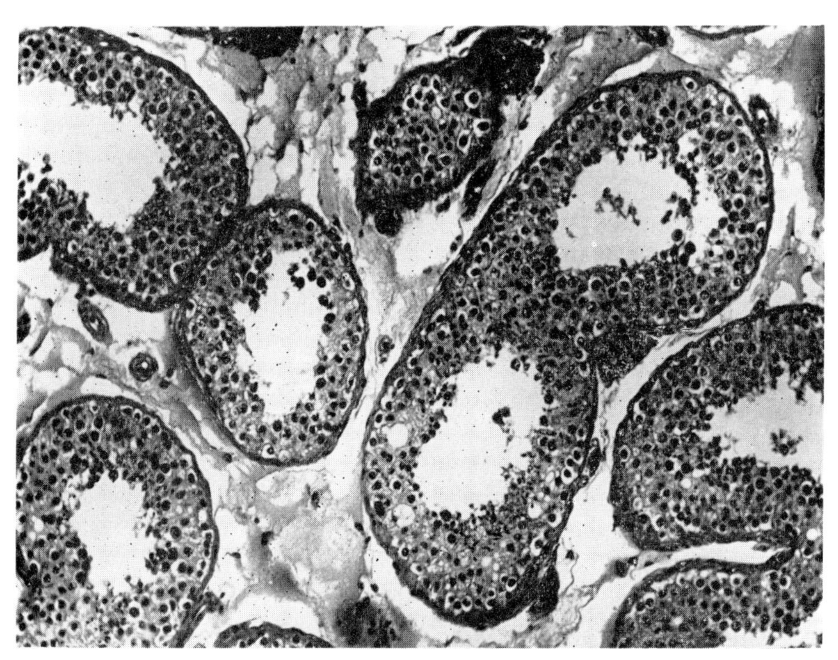

FIG. 4. Photomicrograph of normal testicular biopsy of young adult. The tubules are uniform in size and there is a normal progression of spermatogenesis. The large cells near the thin (normal) basement membrane are spermatogonia. The small black dots extending through the cellular conglomeration to the lumen of the tubules are mature sperm. The interstitial cells of Leydig are demonstrable.

The fetal testis is under the influence of the maternal hormones, to which it strongly reacts. Other hormonal influences are undoubtedly present but as yet have not been confirmed. At birth all maternal influence is suddenly severed and the testis now becomes relatively, but not entirely quiescent. Later the testis becomes active at puberty, when as described above the histologic picture goes through a definite metamorphosis with changes in the tubules and interstitial cells as a result of gonadotropic hormonal stimulation of the pituitary. From here on normal testicular function depends upon normal function of the pituitary and normal responsiveness between the testes and the pituitary gland. Some believe that adrenocortical hormones contribute to the development of the Sertoli cells and normal testicular function. Thus in hyperplasia of the adrenal cortex in young children, one will find tubular enlargement and Sertoli cell maturation without unusual germ cell activity or Leydig cell development.

Sniffen[9, 11, 12] has stressed the fact that the testis in man reacts as a whole and single abnormalities do not occur (with the possible exception of spermatogenesis). He states: "The interstitial cells, the Sertoli cells, and the germ cells are together normal or abnormal. The interstitial cells appear to hold the key position in testicular function, for the tubules are never normal if the Leydig cells are abnormal or absent." This fact suggests that tubular function is dependent, at least in part, on the interstitial cells.

THE NORMAL ADULT TESTIS

The designation "normal testis" is often erroneously used. As a rule it refers to the size, shape and location of the testis under scrutiny. Actually one must include in such a definition the fact that the testis contains seminiferous tubules which proceed and are capable of proceeding to complete cellular maturation with subsequent production of spermatozoa in sufficient amounts for adequate fertility. In addition a normal testis contains Leydig cells which at maturity secrete adequate amounts of androgens for proper development of normal secondary sex characteristics. All of these processes are initiated during puberty as evidenced by the changes in the histological changes of the testes (described above) from birth thru puberty. In adult life the testis assumes its double function: gametogenic and hormonal.

Thus the testis matures for several years after puberty by increasing gametogenic activity and cellular progression. At maturity sperm can be found in most of the tubules at the level of section and various cell types will predominate in different segments of the luminal circumference. Thus, one may find many sperm heads embedded in the Sertoli cytoplasm in one segment and spermatids or spermatocytes at other levels. The gametogenic cells push through the Sertoli cytoplasm which envelops them as they advance toward the lumen apparently by the force exerted by multiple divisions.

For sake of emphasis and for clarification let us now review the characteristic findings as obtained from testicular biopsies and how this knowledge can be applied clinically.

(1) In the normal testicular biopsy, the tubules will be found to be uniform in size. What is most significant is that there is a normal progression of spermatogenesis from the large spermatogonia with their large nucleus, near the thin basement membrane through the mass of the tubule to the lumen, where mature sperm can be seen. The interstitial cells of Leydig are present and appear normal. This type of testicular biopsy can be found in (a) men with normal semen; (b) men with azoospermia but with some ductal obstruction; and (c) not too frequently in men who show normal testicular histology but who still have oligospermia.

(2) Males with complete aspermatogenesis will have sections showing uniform tubules in size and shape but entirely devoid of any wheel and not compressed by the germinal cell. No therapy is indicated in these cases and the biopsy enables the physician to tell the patient immediately that he can stop sterility investigations. Plans for adoption or heterologous artificial insemination are now in order.

(3) In Klinefelter's syndrome the testicular biopsy is of great clinical significance. These cases are usually referred to as progressive tubular sclerosis or sclerosing tubular degeneration and, as the name implies, demonstrate a marked diminution in the number of tubules. Many of the seminiferous tubules are completely destroyed, others are almost obliterated, with marked thickening of the basement membrane. There is no spermatogenic activity whatsoever. There is an unusual amount of normal interstitial cells of Leydig and a widespread thickening of the basement membrane of the tubules. The elastic fibers are decreased in number while the collagenous fibers appear to be increased in number and size. A tremendous amount of hyaline material is seen and the end result

(sclerosis tubular) resembles a small canalized hyaline structure. The fertility in such cases is obviously hopeless and the prognosis for restoring spermatogenesis is as yet poor.

(4) Testicular biopsy is of differential aid in cases of so-called spermatogenic arrest, so aptly described by Engle in which the process of spermatogenesis is arrested at the stage of the primary spermatocyte, with the result that few or no sperm are produced. In this condition the tubules are normal in size with a thickening of the basement membrane. As stated above, the large primary spermatocyte is easily identified. It is the largest cell present with a distinguishable cytoplasm and large distinct nucleus. The arrested cells fragment and slough into the lumen of the tubules. The etiology is obscure.

At one time these cases did not respond to any form of treatment. Heller,[14] Nelson *et al.*, showed that such cases might respond to treatment with testosterone propionate. They obtained testicular biopsies before, during and up to 31 months after treatment. After a course of testosterone propionate, there was decrease in the size of the seminiferous tubules, arrest of spermatogenesis with necrosis of the germinal elements, hyalinization of the basement membrane and tunica propia of the tubules and also disappearance of Leydig cells. What was most significant in this work was that, biopsies of the testis, made at various intervals of time after cessation of treatment, revealed recovery of spermatogenesis and in some patients, the testicular structure was appreciably better than before therapy. Heckel and McDonald[15,17] have studied the effects of testosterone propionate upon the spermatogenic function of the human testis and report a rebound phase, characterized by a striking increase in the number of sperms over that observed prior to treatment. They also report 10 pregnancies, 5 of which resulted in normal healthy babies. Heckel[15] writes, "It would seem, therefore, that the indications for the use of androgens in the treatment of male infertility, are gradually being outlined although there is yet much work to be done in this important field."

The advantage of testicular biopsy in evaluating cryptorchidism is now universally accepted. Charney[16] in a recent communication on the spermatic potential of the undescended testis before and after treatment has resorted to testicular biopsy for "It is the only procedure which accurately reflects existing conditions. Normal size and position of the testis are not necessarily indicative of normal function and the presence of spermatozoa in the ejaculate is significant only in evaluating the result of treatment of bilateral cryptorchism." Thus the data obtained by Charney and others by means of serial testicular biopsies has made possible the following conclusions:

> The testis up to age 9 (resting and growth phase) suffers little damage from its undescended position. At age 10, with initiation of pituitary gonadotropin secretion, a lag in development of the undescended testis is seen. From this time on, the longer the testis remains in the canal, the more marked is the retardation. Such changes as sclerosis and peritubular fibrosis now takes place with accompanying irreversible spermatogenic lesions. What is now even most significant, is that at least 20% of undescended testis are initially hypoplastic, and for this reason alone do not descend, and definitely lack the capacity for normal spermatogenic development. With the initiation of endogenous secretion of pituitary gonadotropins there is further degeneration of the tubular epithelium. A common biopsy finding in adolescent boys who have had orchiopexy performed after the onset of puberty, shows tubules slightly smaller than normal. The tubules may contain spermatogonia but rarely spermatozoa. At times sclerosis and peritubular fibrosis are present. In most instances Leydig cells are present and normal.

The size of the penis in relation to the size of the testicles is often offered as a means of differential diagnosis of sexual precocity due to a cerebral disturbance, adrenal or a gonadal disorder.[21] In sexual precocity of adrenal origin the testicles are small (lack of spermatogenesis) as compared to the obviously enlarged penis; whereas in precocity of cerebral origin or constitutional precocity, spermatogenesis is present and the testicles are enlarged in size proportionate to the size of the penis. Whenever the proportionate relation between the size of the penis and the size of the testicles is not obvious, testicular biopsy serves as a means of identification and diagnosis. It is only by means of a testicular biopsy that the presence or absence of spermatogenesis, as well as the status of the cells of the seminiferous tubules and interstitial tissue can accurately be determined.

Simmons[2] in a study of over 600 testicular biopsies in 100 cases of male sterility attempted a correlation of the semen analysis with testicular biopsy but found it unreliable. From this study it was concluded that from the analysis of the semen, except in cases of complete azoospermia, it is not possible to predict what the testicular biopsy will reveal. Similarly testicular biopsy alone and without other information is no index as to what the semen analysis will reveal.

The senile testis has received considerable attention for many years in the hope that some specific endocrinological factor might be unearthed. Unfortunately no such success has been obtained and because of marked variations in the histological picture of the senile testis no positive statements can be made. Thus in some males, even those who have reached the eighth and ninth decade, testicular biopsy reveals the seminiferous tubules to be fully active and quite comparable to those of younger men. The most common finding is an arrest of spermatogenesis at the primary spermatocyte stage. Sclerosis of the tubules increases with age, with a concomitant thickening of the basement membrane. The Leydig cells like the tubules are also variable in appearance and in many elderly persons the interstitial cells are similar cytologically to those of a young man. Engle[18] describes one specific type of morphological change which occurs with failing spermatogenesis (in the aged). This is the change in the basement membrane and the capsule of the tubule (tunica propria). Under normal circumstances and in the young this is a delicate basement membrane which is surrounded by laminated collagenous and argyrophile fibers. In all tubules of man during the ages of spermatogenesis, this is a thin and delicate membrane providing spermatogenesis is present.[19] In many older people the connective tissue of the tunica propria increases in thickness with a concomitant decrease in the size of the tubule.[20] Generally speaking the ageing process in the male does not leave marked effects on the genital system, as the chronological years influence the genital system in the female.

SUMMARY

(1) Testicular biopsy is a simple procedure of great value in the study of testicular endocrinopathies.

(2) It provides definite information as to the status of the testis.

(3) It eliminates uncertainties in diagnosis.

(4) It aids in evaluating therapy instigated.

REFERENCES

1. Fawcett, D. W., and Burgos, M. H.: Observations on the cytomorphosis of the germinal and interstitial cells of the human testis. *In Ciba Foundation Colloquia on Ageing.* Vol. 2. Ageing in Transient Tissues. Little, Brown and Company, Boston, 1956.
2. Simmons, F. A.: Correlation of Testicular Biopsy Material with Semen Analysis in Male Infertility. *Ann. of the N. Y. Acad. of Sciences 1952,* Vol. 55. Art. 4, part III, 643-656.
3. Charney, C. W.: Testicular Biopsy; Its value in male sterility. *J.A.M.A., 115:* 1429, 1940.
4. Engle, E. T.: The testis biopsy in fertility. *J. Urol., 57:* 789-798, 1947.
5. Hotchkiss, R. S.: *Fertility in Men: A Clinical Study of the Causes, Diagnosis and Treatment of Impaired Fertility in Men.* Lippincott, 1944, Philadelphia.
6. Howard, R. P., Simmons, F. A., and Sniffen, R. C.: Differential Diagnosis in Male Sterility. *J. Fertility and Sterility, 2(2):* 95-114, 1951.
7. Klinefelter, H. F., Jr., Reinfenstein, E. C., Jr., and Albright, F.: Syndrome characterized by gynecomastia, aspermatogenesis without A. leydigism, and increased excretion of follicle stimulating hormone. *J. Clin. Endocrinol., 2:* 615, 1942.
8. Hotchkiss, R. S.: Testicular biopsy in sterility in the male. *Bull. New York Acad. Med., 18,* 600, 1942.
9. Sniffen, R. C., Howard, R. P., and Simmons, F. A.: The Testes: Abnormalities of spermatogenesis and atresia of the excretory ducts. *Arch. Path., 50:* 285, 1950.
10. Charney, C. W., and Wolgin, W.: Cryptorchism. Hoeber-Harper, 1957.
11. Sniffen, R. C.: Histology of the normal and abnormal testis at puberty. *Ann. of the N.Y. Acad. of Sc.,* Vol. 55, p. 609, 1952.
12. Sniffen, R. C.: The Testis. 1. The Normal Testis. *Arch. of Path.,* Vol. 50, p. 259, 1950.
13. Charney, C. W., Conston, A. S., and Meranze, D. R.: Testicular developmental histology. *Ann. of the New York Acad. of Sc.,* Vol. 55, p. 597, 1952.

14. Heller, C. G., Nelson, W. O., Hill, I. B., Henderson, E., Maddocle, W. O., Jungck, E. C., Paulsen, C. A., and Mortimer, G. E.: Improvements in spermatogenesis following depression of the human testis with testosterone. *J. Fertility and Sterility, 1:* 415, 1950.
15. Heckel, M. J., and McDonald, J. H.: Further observations on the rebound phenomenon of the spermatogenic activity of the human testis following the administration of testosterone propionate. *Ann. of the New York Acad. Sc.*, Vol. 55, p. 725-733.
16. Charney, C. W.: The spermatogenic potential of the undescended testis before and after treatment. *J. Urol., 83:* 697, 1960.
17. Heckel, W. J., and McDonald, J. H.: The rebound phenomenon of the spermatogenic activity of the human testis following the administrations of testosterone propionate. *J. Fertility and Steril.*, 3, 49, 1952.
18. Engle, E. T., in Cowdry, E. V., editor: *Problems of Ageing.* Baltimore, Williams and Wilkins Company, 1942.
19. Engle, E. T.: The life history of the human testis. *J. Urol., 74:* 379, 1958.
20. Engle, E. T.: In Conference on problems of ageing. Sponsored by Josiah Macy Jr. Foundation. Endocrine aspects of ageing. New York, 1951.
21. Wershub, L. P.: Testicular biopsy as an aid in diagnosis of testicular endocrinopathies. *J. New York Med. Col. Flower and Fifth Avenue Hospitals, 2:* 33, 1960.
22. Symposium, History of Microscopy–1490 to the Present. *New York State J. Med., 61:* 430-453, 1961.

Chapter 5

THE 17-KETOSTEROIDS

THE URINARY 17-ketosteroids play an important role in the accurate evaluation of many testicular disorders. A basic knowledge of the qualitative patterns of these steroids is essential for the understanding of diseases which are discussed in this book. The nature, origin and significance of the urinary 17-ketosteroids will be analyzed in this chapter.

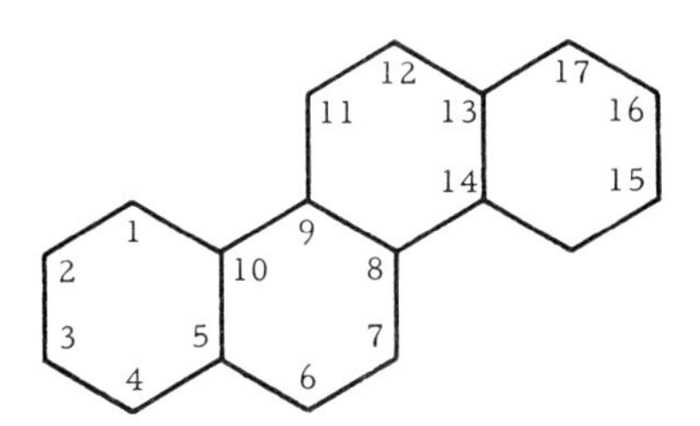

FIG. 5. The steroid nucleus.

The generic term *'steroids'* was first applied to a group of biologically important compounds related to the familiar plant and animal sterols. The bile acids, sex hormones, adrenocortical hormones and the various derivations of these substances, are steroids.[1,2] All have in common a 4 ring nucleus consisting of a cyclopentane ring attached to a hydrogenated phenanthrene ring system and named *cyclopentanoperhydrophenanthrene.* The cyclopentanoperhydrophenanthrene nucleus is the structural arrangement of the naturally occurring sex hormones, including estrogens, progesterone and androgens which are sterols and related chemically to cholesterol and bile acids. Testosterone, produced by the interstitial cells of the testis, is believed to undergo metabolic changes in the liver, as do other steroids, but appear in the urine as active or biologically inactive steroids, the assay of which is used as an index of the androgenic activity of the testis. But what is not known is what percentage of the hormones is lost or used up in the process of its hormonal duties.

What is meant by the term 17-ketosteroids? The term comprises a group of steroid compounds which, as the name indicates, have in common a ketone group at position 17 of the steroid nucleus. All urinary steroids with a ketone group attached in this manner are spoken of as 17-ketosteroids and must not be confused with another fraction of urine containing steroids (corticosteroid fraction). In other words all steroid compounds with a ketone group at position 17 of the steroid nucleus, no matter how they may differ in other structural features, are classified and characterized as neutral 17-ketosteroids. Some of the urinary 17 ketosteroids have androgenic properties but many as etiocholanolone are biologically inactive.

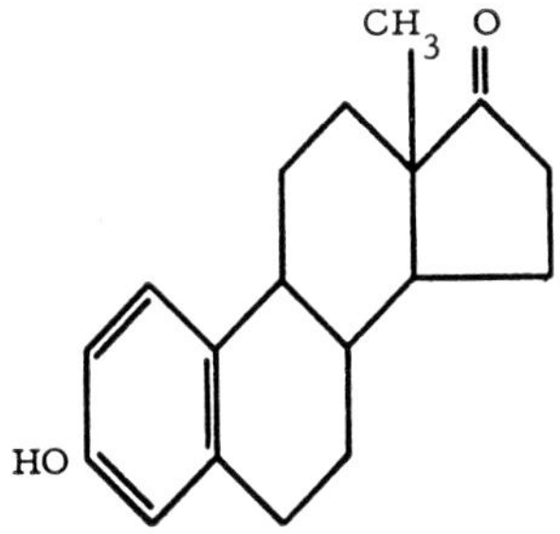

CH_3 O

HO

FIG. 6. Estrone formula.

Estrone is a 17-ketosteroid. It has a phenolic ring, is acidic in nature and thus is removed from the urinary extracts when washed with alkali. It is a 17-ketosteroid but is not classified as a neutral 17-ketosteroid.

The neutral 17-ketosteroids which actually form the urinary products of androgenic metabolism are the end products of substances produced by the *adrenal gland* and the testes. These neutral non-phenolic fractions are divided into alpha and beta ketosteroids. The term alpha and beta refer to the position of the 3-hydroxy group. The neutral 17-ketosteroids are not the only ketosteroids excreted in the urine. As a rule, the alpha fraction makes up the larger percentage of the total neutral ketosteroids excreted in the urine. The beta fraction consists of about 10-15% of the total daily output, although Ronzoni[3] has pointed out that at times greater amounts of beta fractions may be found in normal subjects. As stated elsewhere in the text, the total 17-ketosteroids are increased in the presence of adrenal cortical tumors with a marked increase in the beta fraction in the presence of carcinoma of the adrenal cortex.[4]

Since it is believed that testosterone is manufactured by the human testes, it stands to reason that part of the urinary 17-ketosteroids results from testicular function. It should follow that in cases of testosterone impairment or in cases of absence of the testes there will be a decreased excretion of 17-ketosteroids. Further since normal men excrete, on an average, more 17-ketosteroids than do normal women, men who have destruction of the adrenal cortex (Addison's Disease) may excrete several milligrams of 17-ketosteroids per day, whereas women with the same affliction will excrete negligible amounts of 17-ketosteroids. In fact it has been shown that in the female a destructive lesion of the adrenal cortex practically abolishes the presence of 17-ketosteroids in the urine.

The biological chemist can identify the source of 17-ketosteroids. Thus steroids that have a ketone group at 17, and also oxygenated at position 11 of the steroid nucleus are from the adrenal cortex for only the adrenal cortex is known to produce steroids oxygenated in this position. In addition differences in action depend upon the configuration of the common basic ring system, primarily in position 3, 11 and 17.

Earlier in this chapter reference was made to the corticoid steroids elaborated by the adrenal cortex. Although these steroids can be assayed in the urine, it is well for the reader to bear in mind that the urinary excretion of these steroids does not in any way resemble the urinary excretion of the neutral 17-ketosteroids both in normal and in pathologic states.[5] The neutral 17-ketosteroids are excreted in much larger quantities. The activity of the adrenal corticoids is described in terms of glycogenic units excreted in the urine for twenty-four hours, one glycogenic unit being equivalent to the biologic activity of one microgram of 17-hydroxy-11-dehydrocorticosterone. Like the neutral 17-ketosteroids, the excretion of the corticoids is somewhat higher in normal males than in females. They are present in very small amounts in the newborn infant but rapidly increases in its secretory rate so that by two and one-half years normal adult levels are reached. The average adult normal range for males varies from 40 to 85 glycogenic units per twenty-four hours, while for females the range varies between 25 and 55 units. Soffer[5] states, "These values are markedly reduced in Addison's disease and in pan-hypopituitarism and are only slightly, if at all, reduced in anorexia nervosa. In Cushing's syndrome they are generally markedly elevated, frequently attaining a value of several hundred. Physiologic states such as pregnancy, particularly late pregnancy and muscular exercise are accompanied by an increased excretion of the corticoids. Essentially the same is true following trauma, infection and surgical procedures. In short, any state associated with an increase in adrenal cortical function will cause an increase in the manufacture and excretion of the glycogenic corticoids."

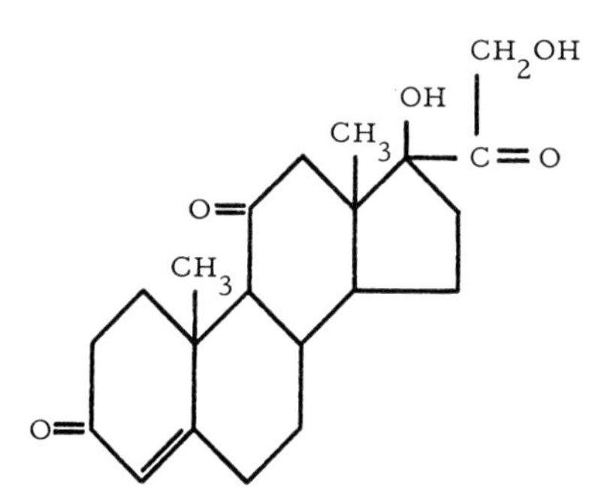

FIG. 7. Cortisone formula.

The above arrangement represents a cortical steroid, 11-dehydro-17-hydroxycorticosterone, also known as cortisone and as compound E of Kendall. In general such steroids with a common oxygenation at position 11, in the forms of carbonyl or an hydroxl group are mainly concerned with catabolism of protein and glucogenesis and not with gonadal function (see section on Testes and the Adrenals).

Steroids with androgen, estrogen and progentational actions have been isolated from the adrenal gland. The estrogen and progestional actions of these steroids are relatively weak, and quantitatively make up only a small percentage of the total steroids manufactured by the adrenal cortex. Of singular interest is that in adrenocortical hyperplasia and neoplasia, feminizing changes may occur and under such circumstances the urinary estrogens are increased. Androgens which are derived from the adrenal cortex appear to be associated with muscular vigor and with the growth of axillary and pubic hair.

In normal subjects adrenocortical activity is responsible for two-thirds of the 17-ketosteroid excretion in the male and for the total excretion of urinary 17-ketosteroids in the female. As will be discussed later, the excretion of urinary 17-ketosteroids is considered to be an index of the androgenic activity of the testes and the adrenal cortex. To be emphasized is that urinary 17-ketosteroids include biologically active androgens and inactive androgen-like substances. Testosterone is a most potent androgen but is not a 17-ketosteroid. Urinary ketosteroids are believed to be the end products of androgen secretion by the adrenal cortex.

It has recently been postulated that the cortical hormone itself is broken down in the liver and other tissues of the body to 17-ketosteroids. Sayers[6] and others[13] have advocated that urinary 17-ketosteroids output should be rejected as an index of adrenocortical activity, not because of the uncertainty of its physiological significance but because of the lack of correlation between the rate of 17-ketosteroids excretion and adrenocortical activity. Forbes *et al.*,[7] Venning and Browne,[8] quoted by Sayers,[6] interpret the lack of parallelism between the rate of excretion of 17-ketosteroids and corticoids as evidence in support of a dual function of the adrenal cortex. Thus 17-ketosteroid excretion is taken as an index of the androgenic activity of the adrenal cortex, and corticoids as an index of the rate of secretion of cortical hormone. These authors attribute the reduction of 17-ketosteroids with stress to mean that the androgenic activity of the gland has been reduced and that cortical hormone secretion has gained precedence to meet an emergency. The interested reader is referred to the review of Sayers[6] for a more detailed discusison of the adrenal cortex.

The reader may well ask, "What are the normal values of 17-ketosteroids?" Mason and Engstrom[9] point out that, "With one or two exceptions there is a general agreement that the values for the 17-ketosteroids excreted by normal young adult men and women cover a wide range and that there is considerable overlapping in the values of the two sexes. However, there is considerable disagreement as to the lower and upper limits of this range and the mean values." These authors stress that the disagreements may be attributed in part to the limited number of individual studies made in many instances, and in part to the different methods used. They recommend that each laboratory, whenever practical, set up its standards of normal values. In all instances there is a great variation in output of 17-ketosteroids in normal adults. The rate of excretion is not constant in 24 hours, or even from day to day. Pincus[10] quoted by Mason and Engstrom,[9] observed that the rate of excretion of 17-ketosteroids was higher during the day than during the night. Although the rate of formation of urine during sleep was less, forced diuresis in one subject did not significantly alter the excretion of 17-ketosteroids.

The exact relationship between volumes of urine and excretion of 17-ketosteroids has not as yet been defined. Actually in view of the many physiologic variables which may affect the excretion of 17-ketosteroids, ordinary variations in the volume of urine probably plays no significant role in 17-ketosteroid production. Since there are, however, discrepancies between the diurnal and nocturnal titers it is advised that the urine should be collected over a 24-hour period, even though a longer period would give a more accurate picture of the excretion of 17-ketosteroids.

In the normal healthy male, values up to 27 mg. of 17-ketosteroids have been found to be excreted in the urine per day. Males normally secrete on an average more 17-ketosteroids than do normal women. It has been estimated that average values are 14 mg. per 24 hours for men and 9 mg. for women. It is believed that the average difference of 5 mg. represents the amount from the testes (9 mg. believed to originate in the adrenal cortex of the male and female). In this matter, Scott and Hudson[11] state, "whereas it seems reasonably clear that the testes and the adrenal cortex are responsible for these steroids, their precursors in these organs are poorly understood. Some clinicians have considered the urinary 17-ketosteroids to be an index of androgenic activity of these structures, but it must again be emphasized that all urinary 17-ketosteroids are not biological androgens." "It will be clear," continue these authors, "that the determination of total urinary 17-ketosteroids and the beta-fraction are of considerable importance as laboratory aids in the diagnosis of certain disorders of the testes and adrenals, it would appear at present that their output is not a sensitive measure of changing rates of secretion of cortical hormone by the adrenal cortex in man, particularly over a short period of time."

When studies of 17-ketosteroids were made of older people, lowered values of 17-ketosteroids excretion, suggested diminished testicular and adrenal cortical production of steroid hormones.

Data on the excretion of 17-ketosteroids of children from early childhood to late puberty have revealed no significant differences. Indeed there is little difference of steroid excretion of the two sexes up to 18 years of age. Mason and Engstrom[9] believe that excretion of 17-ketosteroids by children up to 6 or 8 years is likely to be slight and frequently less than one mg. per day. In both boys and girls this amount increases slowly to the age of puberty. After puberty it is greater for boys than for girls and the average adult levels are approached but not reached until approximately 17 years of age. Talbot[12] and his associates believe that by 12 years of age, the child should excrete about 1 mg. of 17-ketosteroids per day. Of singular interest is that during childhood the equivalent amounts of urinary 17-ketosteroids excreted by boys and girls suggest that the source during childhood is from the adrenal cortex.

The 17-ketosteroids are markedly influenced by specific changes in the endocrine glands. Thus a pathologic process involving the pituitary, thyroid, testes, ovaries or adrenal cortex will show marked fluctuations in the amounts of 17-ketosteroids excreted. We will confine our discussion to pathological changes in the pituitary, testes and adrenal cortex.

Since gonadal function is under pituitary control, it follows that pituitary insufficiency would be associated with a marked decrease of 17-ketosteroids in either male or female. Sufficient evidence has been accumulated to show that the function of the adrenal cortex as well as the testes is directly controlled by a trophic hormone produced by the anterior pituitary gland. Injection of this hormone (ACTH)) produces an increase in the amount of cortico-steroids excreted. A tumor of the anterior pituitary gland, as for example chromophobe adenomas, produce endocrine disturbances since they interfere with the normal function of the gland. Excretion of 17-ketosteroids in these cases vary. In some cases there is an increase and in others a decrease in the excretion of 17-ketosteroids.

As stated above the interstitial cells of Leydig produce androgens (testosterone) which contribute to the excretion of urinary 17-ketosteroids. It would seem that failure of these cells to function properly would produce a reduction in the excretion of 17-ketosteroids. Yet it has been clinically demonstrated, that even with complete failure of the cells of Leydig to function, by either atrophy or degeneration, that there is no appreciable decrease in the 24-hour excretions of 17-ketosteroids. The genesis of failure to decrease the excretion of 17-ketosteroids under such circumstances has as yet not been entirely explained. As will be discussed in later chapters of this book, a deficiency of testicular function that exists and originates prior to puberty may not produce the same effect on the excretion of 17-ketosteroids, as a deficiency of testicular function that occurs at puberty. A normal reading for excretion of urinary 17-ketosteroids does not rule out failure of manufacture of testosterone by the testes. A low reading for excretion of urinary 17-ketosteroids does not indicate a primary gonadal failure although it should arouse suspicion of testicular dysgenesis. Where the levels are above normal or within normal range, the source of the urinary 17-ketosteroids is believed to be the adrenal cortex. Indeed this may be the underlying explanation of increased production of 17-ketosteroids after castration.

As in disturbances of the testicle, certain disturbances of the adrenal cortex will reflect itself in either an abnormally high or low excretion of 17-ketosteroids. Since the same clinical picture may be found in either neoplasia or hyperplasia of the adrenal cortex, it is often difficult to distinguish between these two entities. Evaluation of the urinary 17-ketosteroids may be of some help in the differential diagnosis, but the reader must bear in mind that often the results are equivocal. As will be discussed in the chapter on the adreno-genital syndrome, adrenal hyperplasia is usually characterized by low total 17-ketosteroids in the urine whereas when tumor (carcinoma) is present there is usually marked elevation of total urinary 17-ketosteroids.

An important difference, stressed by Mason and Engstrom,[9] between the composition of the 17-ketosteroid fraction in the urine of patients with cortical hyperplasia and those with cortical tumor is the preponderance of dehydroisoandrosterone in the urine of patients with tumor. The significance of dehydroisoandrosterone in relation to the adrenal cortex is still not completely understood. Since it has been recovered in the urine of patients without adrenal disease it appears likely that it is a product of normal adrenal cortical function. On the other hand it may be a product of the adrenal cortex produced in abnormal quantities by a tumor, or it may be a by-product of some reaction or the end product of some unidentified precursor.

In order to make the story complete a word about the role of 17-ketosteroids as an aid in differential diagnosis of intersex follows: In female pseudohermaphroditism there is an excessive production of androgens caused by hyperplasia of the adrenal cortex. In such patients the gonads are ovaries but the external genitalia and sexual characteristics are more or less masculine. A male pseudohermaphrodite is an individual whose gonads are testes but whose external genitalia and sexual characteristics are more or less female. In female hermaphroditism (caused by congenital adrenal hyperplasia) the value of urinary neutral 17-ketosteroids is consistently elevated. Thus if we accept the normal value for adult females to be about 8 mg. per 24 hours, values from 25-100 mg./24 hours for total neutral 17-ketosteroids should arouse suspicion of the underlying condition associated with the general clinical picture of abnormal sexual characteristics.

Since the disorder should be suspected in childhood as well as after puberty, the reader must bear in mind that most female children under 2 years of age normally excrete less than 1 mg. per day, and that from 2-8 years of age, values up to 2 mg. per day may be accepted as normal.* From 8 years of age to puberty the value increases and approaches the normal adult reading. Interestingly enough one notes that in progressive virilization of female hermaphroditism due to adrenal hyperplasia the estrogenic secretion of these patients is high and not low as would be expected. Thus the biologic effect of the estrogenic influence is neutralized by excessive androgen formation and further estrogens found here are of adrenal origin and not gonadal.

The differentiation is greatly aided by the so-called suppression test in which the excess androgens are suppressed by the administration of cortisone. In the adult or the older child, where it is also indicated, 100 mg. of cortisone is given daily for 3-7 consecutive days. If the pseudohermaphroditism is the result of congenital adrenal hyperplasia there will be a marked drop in the amount of urinary 17-ketosteroids on the 3rd to 7th day of the test; whereas if due to cortical tumor there will be no drop in the urinary 17-ketosteroids; in fact there actually may be an increase in the urinary 17-ketosteroids. When suppression does take place, the reduction is approximately two-thirds of the pre-test level.

As stated above a male pseudohermaphrodite is an individual whose gonads are testes but whose external genitalia and secondary sexual characteristics are more or less feminine. For normal masculine development a normally functioning testis is essential. In male hermaphroditism the basic disorder is invariably one of anatomical abnormal and physiologically abnormal testes. Endocrine studies in these cases of intersexuality have been interesting but variable and particularly not enlightening since investigations of the urinary 17-ketosteroids has only been made on a

---

*It should be noted that the critical determination of hermaphroditism, in the *new born,* is that of the urinary 17-ketosteroids. If these are elevated the diagnosis must be either (a) congenital adrenal hyperplasia; or (b) adrenal tumor. Adrenal tumor is rarely if ever seen in the new born, but does occur in older children as well as in adults. Wilkins survey up to 1948 reveals no tumors responsible for this syndrome in the new born.

limited number of such persons. Some reports reveal urinary 17-ketosteroid levels at or slightly above that reported for normal females. Estrogen levels have been reported at normal or below adult levels. Where fractionation of the 17-ketosteroids was done it showed low levels due to low levels of andosterone and etiochanolane. This is of singular interest, since these metabolites are believed to be mainly of testicular origin and would therefore confirm the clinical impression of poor testicular function.

It is unfortunate that in feminizing adrenal cortical tumors in males the relationship of urinary levels of 17-ketosteroids has not as yet been universally applied. In the few instances it has been investigated, the work has been more or less limited to the so-called total neutral 17-ketosteroids. Most researchers now believe such investigations should include fractionation of the alpha and beta components. Indeed Mason and Engstrom[9] believe that a daily excretion of more than 50 mg. of 17-ketosteroids, 50% or more of which is beta fraction, should suggest the presence of an adrenal cortical tumor. As stated before high values of urinary 17-ketosteroids suggest malignant tumor whereas non-elevation or slightly elevated or even below normal are more suggestive of adreno-cortical hyperplasia or a simple benign tumor.

SUMMARY

(1) Estimation of the total neutral 17-ketosteroid excretion gives an index of the androgenic activity of the adrenal cortex and testes and gross variations from the normal give some clue as to the underlying etiology of the disturbance.

(2) The urinary neutral 17-ketosteroid normal values are somewhat higher in men than in women. The difference actually being 5 mgms, undoubtedly the amount of neutral 17-ketosteroids manufactured by the male gonads.

(3) The 17-ketosteroids progressively increases from childhood up to the age of 40, and then begins to decrease. From age 4 to 7 years of age, 1.3 mg. per 24 hours, represents the average urinary output of children. From the age of 7 to 12, 4.0 mg.; from 12 to 15, 8.2 mg.; adult female, 10.2; and adult male 15.0 mg.

(4) The urinary excretion of the neutral 17-ketosteroids varies with different pathologic states: In hyperfunctions of the adrenal cortex there is a definite increase and the highest levels are seen in adrenal cortical carcinoma. In this disease the neutral urinary 17-ketosteroids may reach over 60 mgm. per 24 hours. In patients exhibiting signs of virilism but without definite cortical pathology, the urinary 17-ketosteroids may be normal or only slightly increased, in post-puberal patients. When virilism occurs before puberty, the urinary excretion of neutral 17-ketosteroids is usually increased either moderately or considerably. Patients with Cushing's syndrome but without demonstrative cortical changes excrete normal amounts of the neutral 17-ketosteroids. In cortical hyperplasia with symptoms of Cushing's syndrome there is slight to moderate increases in the urinary excretion of neutral 17-ketosteroids.

(5) In cases of cortical tumor removal, or other disturbances therapeutically ameliorated, there occurs a rapid decrease in the excretion of neutral urinary 17-ketosteroids.

(6) In adrenal cortical carcinoma the increase in urinary 17-ketosteroids is mainly demonstrated by increase in the excretion of the beta ketosteroids. The alpha 17-ketosteroids are elaborated both by the adrenal cortex and by the male gonads, whereas the beta ketosteroids (isoandrosterone and dehydroisoandrosterone) presumably arise from the adrenal cortex. Under normal circumstances 10-20% of the total neutral 17-ketosteroids are made up of the beta fraction. Dehydroisoandrosterone is the main ingredient of the beta fractions found in the urine and it is with very few exceptions greatly increased in the presence of a malignant adrenal cortical tumor and rarely elevated in the presence of a benign cortical tumor or in bilateral adrenal cortical hyperplasia.

(7) Cortico-steroids should not be confused with 17-ketosteroids. The former are purely an end product of the adrenal cortex.

REFERENCES

1. Callow, R. K.: Excretion of sex hormones in urine. *Proc. Roy. Soc. Med., 31:* 841, 1938.
2. Callow, N. H., and Callow, R. K.: Isolation of 17-ketosteroids from urine of normal women. *Biochem. J., 33:* 931, 1939.

3. Ronzoni, E.: Excretion of dehydroisoandresterone during adrenal stimulation with adrenocorticotropic hormone. *J. Clin. Endrocrin. and Metab., 12:* 517, 1952.
4. Frazer, R. W., Forbes, A. P., Albright, F., Sulkowitch, H., and Reifenstein, E. C., Jr.: Colormetric assay of 17-ketosteroids in urine. *J. Clin. Endocrin., 1:* 234, 1931.
5. Soffer, L. J.: in Sohval, A. R.: *Diseases of the Endocrine Glands.* Section 3. The Gonads. Lea and Febiger, Philadelphia. 2nd Edition, 1958.
6. Sayers, G.: The adrenal cortex and hemeostasis. *Physio. Rev.,* Vol. 30, No. 3, July, 1950.
7. Forbes, A. B., and Albright, F.: Adrenal Hormones. *J. Clin. Endocrinol., 11:* 926, 1951.
8. Venning, E. H., Hoffman, M. M., and Browne, J. S. L.: The Adrenal steroids: *Endocrinology, 35:* 49, 1944.
9. Mason, H. L., and Engstrom, W. W.: 17-Ketosteroids; their origin, determination and significance. *Physiol. Rev., 30:* 321-374, 1950.
10. Pincus, G., Hechter, O., and Zaffaroni, A.: Effect of ACTH upon steroid genesis by the isolated perfused adrenal gland, Proc. 2nd clinical ACTH Conference, Vol. 1, 40, 1950. Blakiston Co., Philadelphia.
11. Scott, W. W., and Hudson, P. B.: *Surgery of the Adrenal Glands.* Thomas, Springfield, 1954.
12. Talbot, N. B., Butler, A. M., and Mac Lachan, E. A.: Alpha and beta neutral ketosteroids (Androgens), *New England J. Med.,* 223, 369, 1940.
13. Jones, H. W., Jr., and Scott, W. W. *Hermaphroditism, Genital Anomalies and Related Endocrine Disorders.* Baltimore, The Williams and Wilkins Company, 1958.

Chapter 6

CHROMOSOMES AND CHROMATIN SEX

WITHIN THE PAST few years several unusual and interesting improvements in cellular studies have been made so that researchers can now investigate the ultra structure of chromosomes. This has given rise to new theories; many of which await further confirmation. Chromatin sex is one of the outcomes of such investigations and one which has been confirmed by clinical data.[1, 2, 3, 4, 5, 6]

For many years it was a universally accepted fact that human beings had 48 chromosomes. Subsequently the number was 46 and now some researchers have reported the number as 47. More intensive studies have led to the characterization of these chromosomes based on their size, position of centromere and possession of a satellite.*

These techniques, in turn, have enabled the clinician to classify certain sexual anomalies. For example, studies have revealed that the genotype of persons with Klinefelter's and Turner's syndrome differ from the normal sex chromosome pattern of XX in the female and XY in the male. Studies are also under way which tend to confirm the belief that persons with Turner's syndrome (ovarian agenesis) have an XO chromosomal pattern rather than an XY configuration. Similarly, those with Klinefelter's syndrome (testicular dysgenesis) are found to have an XXY chromosomal pat-

---

*In 1956, Ford and Hamerton,[5] and Tjo and Levan[7] definitely established the normal human chromosome number to be 46. This number denotes 22 pairs of autosomes and 2 sex chromosomes, paired in the female (XX) and unpaired in the male (XY). Within recent years many reports have appeared in the literature concerning chromosomal aberrations. Such reports are confined to definite pathologic conditions in which abnormal numbers of chromosomes are reported as definite deviations from the normal human diploid number of 46.

tern.* Of course, these generalizations are not final, and they must await confirmation by further studies. The rapid changes in our modern concept of cellular chromosomes is further exemplified by the report[12] from England of the so-called "super female" with an XXX chromosome pattern (positive identification of the third X chromosome is not accepted by all workers.) This woman was quite normal in appearance except for slightly undeveloped primary and secondary sexual characteristics; menstruation commenced at 14 and stopped at 19; at surgical exploration (aged 28) the ovaries were found to be post menopausal; buccal smear cells showed many chromatin bodies. No reports of a YO pattern have been made. It should be noted that the presence of X chromosome seems to be a prerequisite for some essential enzyme systems.

It can at least be said that individuals may possess chromosomes and genetic traits quite different from the normal pattern and that by means of special techniques these chromosome patterns can be detected. Such is the pattern in sexual anomalies as Turner's syndrome, Klinefelter's syndrome, mongolism, adrenogenital syndrome, testicular feminization, male and female pseudo-hermaphroditism and true hermaphroditism. In all these disorders genetic factors are the underlying influence or basic cause in the development of the sexual anomaly. Where normal sexual development takes place changes may *subsequently* occur which can influence the interaction between the somatic tissue and hormones. This may be the result of either: (1) faulty synthesis of a specific hormone; or (2) change in the responsiveness of the tissue.

It is known that in most species, the sex chromosomes contain conspicuous masses of heterochromatin. In a few species of insects, the heterochromatin persists in the intermitotic nucleus

---

*Thus, in mongolism a chromosome number of 47 with trisomy for one of the smallest acrocentric autosomes have been reported. Deviation of the chromosome number to 47 in Klinefelter's syndrome has also been reported.[9] This deviation is attributed to the combination of 3 sex chromosomes (XXY). Patients with Turner's syndrome (gonadal dysgenesis) have been reported with a chromosome number of 45 because of the presence of only a single sex-determining chromosome, resulting in an XO sex chromosome pattern.[10, 11]

as a characteristic chromatin mass or masses. These masses are sufficiently characteristic to distinguish the nuclei of male from those of female insects. That similar sex differences might be demonstrated in the more refactory nuclei of mammals was not supposed until Barr[13] and Bertram in 1949 demonstrated this difference in the nerve cells of the hypoglossal nucleus of the cat. Thus one of the most unusual and revealing techniques, based upon sex differences in nuclear morphology of various cells, became available. This procedure first reported by Moore, Graham and Barr[25] in 1953 has revolutionized many of the formerly held concepts of certain testicular endocrinopathies.

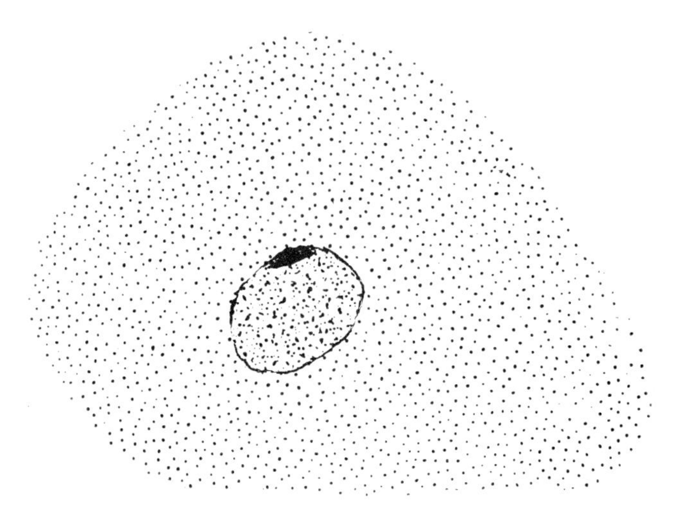

FIG. 8. Oral mucosal smear in case of Klinefelter's syndrome. Nucleus shows typical mass of sex chromatin adjacent to nuclear membrane.

The test is based upon the detection or absence of "nucleolar satellites" in somatic cells but it must not be accepted as foolproof and the final criterion for sex determination. Indeed, Barr[14] has stated, "It is premature to equate female-type nuclei with genetic femaleness or male-type nuclei with genetic maleness, as a generalization in errors of sex development, for our present methods give no direct information concerning the genes that are concerned with sex determination and sex differentiation." Lennox[15] on the other hand states, "the best answer to doubts as to the complete validity of the method is the fact that, although thousands of tests have been done, no normal fertile human being has yet been reported whose nuclear sex does not correspond to his or her apparent sex, the subject proves to have some disorder of sexual development."*

This method of nuclear sexing has been of tremendous value in the diagnosis of certain abnormalities but its true significance has yet to be fully worked out. Thus it is difficult to say to what extent 'sex' abnormalities occur as a result of genetic factors affecting the sex chromosomes or the role of endocrine factors early (fetal) and late in life. It is for this reason that in true hermaphrodites where the nuclear findings are sometimes confusing, that these abnormalities are best classified according to histology of the gonad. From this and subsequent discussion, it is obvious that though the nuclear chromatin pattern and the morphologic character of the gonads are important, neither can be used alone as the criterion in which to decide the sex in which a child should be reared, for it can never be said with certainty whether subsequent secondary sexual development will be masculine or feminine.

The sex chromatin body as described by Barr and his associates[16] is as follows: As is well known the human female carries in each cell two similar sex chromosomes, XX. The male carries one X and a smaller chromosome Y. In most cells of normal females, a sex chromatin body (often referred to as the chromatin "blob," mass, or clump, or nuclear satellite) is found in cell nuclei on or very close to the nuclear membrane. This formation is believed to be derived from certain regions of the two chromosomes in opposition. Thus it is possible on a basis of cytological classification to identify patients as either belonging to one group, chromatin positive (female) or to another group, chromatin negative (male). When the majority of cell nuclei in a tissue show the sex

*In a later communication Barr definitely confirms the use of the "tests of chromosomal sex" and points out that the basis for this is the existence of sexual dimorphism in the structure of intermitotic nuclei in man and certain other mammals. The difference in the sexes being a special mass of sex chromatin clearly visible in the nuclei of normal females but not in those of normal males.

chromatin body, the specimen is said to be chromatin positive, and when as in the male, the sex chromatin body is not observed or only seen in few numbers, the specimen is said to be chromatin negative. The sex of an individual evaluated in this manner is referred to as the "chromatin sex."

Sex chromatin is characteristic of nuclei in females. "It usually adheres to the inner surface of the nuclear membrane. It is about 1 mm in diameter, has an affinity for basic dyes, reacts positively to tests for desoxyribonucleic acid, stains readily with the Feulgen technique and with methyl green and can be identified in 60-80% of nuclei. The presence of sex chromatin in the tests of chromosomal sex means only that the nuclei contain heterochromatin regions of the 2X chromosomes. One chromosome may be defective in its euchromatic region, there may be an unusual sex chromatin complex (such as XXY) or the autosomes that bear the male determiners may be in some way abnormal. Conversely, absence of sex chromatin in the tests of chromosomal sex indicates only that 2 normal X chromosomes are not present. The sex chromosome constitution could be XO or there could be an abnormality of the autosomes carrying male determiners."*[16]

---

*Shortly after Barr introduced his technique for nuclear sexing, it became apparent that many patients with Klinefelter's syndrome were chromatin positive, but that many who had been classified as having Klinefelter's syndrome were chromatin-negative. This paradoxical problem has aroused much speculation. Stewart and his workers have divided their cases into the chromatin-positive and the chromatin-negative types and demonstrated that there may be uniform phenotypic and pathological differences between the two groups, although a sharp demarcation is not obvious. Thus patients with this affliction and with chromatin-positive tend more to the eunuchoid group, and those with chromatin-negative are phenotypically masculine.

More recently Jacobs and Strong[9] have demonstrated that patients with Klinefelter's syndrome, and chromatin-positive, have an XXY pattern of the chromosomes. These authors believe the extra sex chromosome arises during the first or perhaps the second mitotic division by nondisjunction of the sex chromosomes.

In the chromatin-negative group, Yerganian[17] and his group believes that there are two kinds of X chromosome and that the pattern in Klinefelter's syndrome, whether in the chromatin-positive or chromatin-negative, depends upon the pattern of the different X-chromosomes with which the particular patient is endowed.

Stanbury[18] and others point out that the difficulty with this formulation is that it postulates 3 sex chromosomes in both chromatin-positive and chromatin-negative patients with the syndrome. "It is possible," states Stanbury, "that the chromatin-negative group is monosomic for an autosome and trisomic for the sex chromosomes. In these studies the sex chromosomes are identified only morphologically, and there is ample opportunity for error."

Although sex chromatin is present in all somatic tissues, many types of cells with nuclei which are either too small or too dense are excluded for use in diagnosing genetic sex. Thus certain cells because of large nuclei and ready availability are used more frequently. The buccal tissue[19] and vaginal smear method are the most convenient areas utilized. In the buccal smear method, smears are prepared by scraping the mucosa of the cheek with the edge of a narrow metal spatula, transferring the material to a slide, and fixing and staining with a basic dye. By this technique one finds in normal females, 20 to 79% of the nuclei in the cells of the buccal scraping to contain visible sex chromatin bodies. In males, smears of the same technique show these bodies in less than 4 percent of the nuclei.

Vaginal[20] epithelium, whenever available, is usually the best source for study of chromatin sex in women. The vesicular nuclei of pre-cornified epithelial cells found in such smears reveal sex chromatin bodies in as many as 97 to 98% of the nuclei if a special staining technique is utilized.

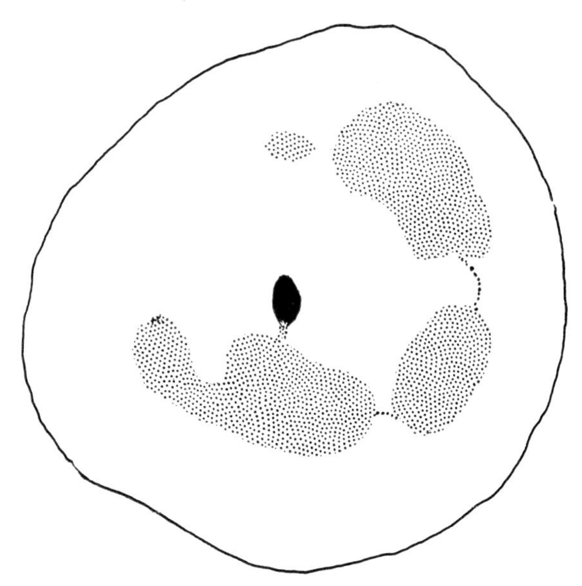

FIG. 9. White blood cell with female phenotype chromatin pattern; demonstrating so called "drum-stick"; taken from case of Klinefelter's syndrome.

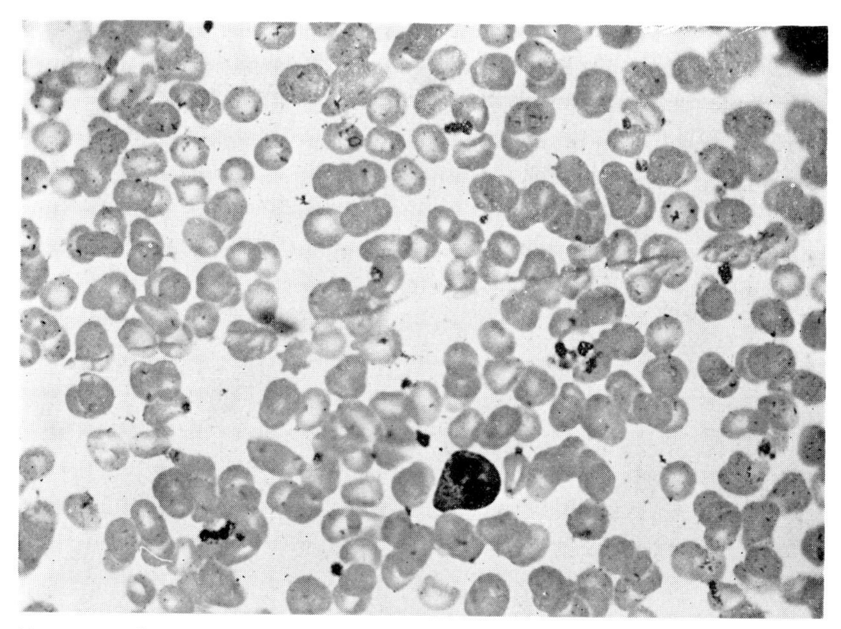

FIG. 10. Photomicrograph of blood smear with female chromatin pattern (case of Klinefelter's syndrome). Typical pattern well demonstrated at six o'clock, with two very large chromcenters within the cell.

The neutrophil procedure[21] is based on sexual dimorphism in the nuclei of neutrophil leukocytes. In women, a small proportion of neutrophils (2-3%) has an accessory nuclear lobule, called a "drumstick," that is lacking in neutrophils of males. Some believe that the drumstick contain the sex chromatin body, but there is no general agreement on this point. Because of the small number of positive cells, at least 500 neutrophils must be examined before a patient may be declared chromatin negative.

Chromosome preparations may be obtained from biopsy specimens of bone marrow and have been used in studying Klinefelter's syndrome. Ford[20] and his associates used this technique to study three patients with Klinefelter's syndrome. One was chromatin positive, one chromatin negative and one chromatin positive with an unexpected result because detailed analysis of the chromosome pattern showed 47 chromosome cells that contained XXY, twelve of which were studied in detail. All contained

5 short acrocentric chromosomes plus 16 chromosomes in the medium-length group (as in a female). The other ten chromosomes were the 5 long pairs common to both sexes. This was interpreted by the authors as the cells containing 2X chromosomes and 1Y chromosome beside the normal 22 pairs of autosomes. However, the possibility that they are basically female and trisomic for one of the small acrocentric autosomes is not excluded (see footnote on preceding page).

The chromatin sex test is of great value in making a decision as to the sex of an inter sex child at birth, without recourse to surgery.[22, 23, 24] In such instances the decision can be made at an early age and proper rearing, training and education inaugurated. Of course it is not entirely infallible, and special circumstances may alter such decisions despite the interpretation of the chromatin sex pattern. (See section on sex and its determination.)

Of singular importance is the clear appreciation, that these new chromosomal techniques have not only altered the handling of these patients but they have widened the theoretical understanding of these sexual abnormalities. In all instances what is apparent is that these disorders imply that genetic factors influence development in various ways. Thus changes may occur because of certain influences during fetal development, particularly at the time when the undifferentiated gonadal tissue is being influenced towards a particular sex development. Even after sexual characteristics (anatomically) are developed, influences between the somatic tissues and hormones may occur. Regardless of the cause, the phase or degree of influence, the result is a distinct medical problem.

Lennox,[22] Serr and Ferguson-Smith state the possible applications of nuclear sexing are numerous and not confined to the study of intersexes:

(1) It is immediately applicable in diagnosis of variations of sex in early life. Most practical is the recognition of congenital adrenal virilism in female infants, for in such cases the utilization of cortisone both reverses the virilization and eliminates a great risk of death from adrenocortical failure. These authors state, "Because adrenal virilization is the only common cause of

masculinoid genital malformation in female infants, all infants of doubtful sex at birth should be sexed (by oral mucosal smear usually), and in all cases found to be female by this method the adrenal cortex may be assumed to be at fault till proven to be otherwise."

(2) Nuclear sexing tests are of value in sex reversals. Such cases as the chromatin-negative (genetic male) feminoids of Turner's syndrome, the chromatin-positive (genetic female) masculinoids of Klinefelter's syndrome, and the genetic male (testicular feminization, Petterson and Bonmier syndrome) fall into this category of available aid in differential diagnosis.

(3) Tumors usually have the nuclear sex of their hosts, except in cases of teratomata and chorionepithelioma. Such variations also occur in other anaplastic tumors.

(4) In addition to such practical uses, sex chromatin studies are advantageous for further evaluation of the genetic material in the so-called "resting nucleus." This undoubtedly requires further study and clarification in an attempt to contribute more data to this subject.

The clinical use of the chromatin sex test cannot be underestimated in problems of infertility. Thus the finding of a chromatin sex pattern opposite to that of the anatomic sex means an irreparable sterile patient. For example the finding in an overt female, of a chromatin-negative pattern (male) means the absence of gonadal tissue or the inability of whatever gonadal tissue is present, to produce a gamate. In like fashion, a chromatin-positive pattern (female) in an overt male, implies sterility. Under such circumstances there is no need for further physiologic or anatomic investigations to determine the underlying cause of infertility.

The early diagnosis of dysgenesis of the seminiferous tubules (Klinefelter's syndrome) is now possible by means of the chromatin sex test. This disorder was seldom diagnosed before puberty but since it has now been shown that the majority of males with this disorder have chromatin-positive nuclei, the disease is now more readily recognized at an earlier age. Although the thought of sterility is of no immediate concern during childhood, early diagnosis and proper management may ultimately prevent serious complications in untreated adult cases. Klinefelter's syndrome may also exist in a chromatin-negative male child.

The recent development of tissue culture methods for human cells and improved techniques for the determination of the number and morphology of mammalian chromosomes have made possible the accumulation, within a period of a few years, of a large amount of data, which have established the normal diploid number of chromosomes in human somatic cells[17, 18] as 46. This number comprises 22 pairs of autosomes and two sex chromosomes (XX in the female and XY in the male).

It is suggested that such studies be continued and the chromosomal pattern of parents and siblings be investigated wherever possible. The accumulation of such data on a large scale should be of great help not only on the classification and better understanding of such disorders, but also aid the geneticist in the identification of the hereditary nature of such conditions.

Although we are not concerned with Mongolism in our dissertation it would not be amiss to point out that recent investigations of the chromosome count in Mongolism has been most significant. Thus patients with Mongolism have been shown to have an extra chromosome. A study of somatic chromosomes in six typical Mongolian idiots were consistent with their apparent sex and in all cases, the chromosome count was 47; the extra chromosome was evidently one of the smallest autosomes rather than a sex chromosome. An interesting male patient has been reported, with both Klinefelter's syndrome and Mongolism.[27] In this case, an extra X chromosome and an extra autosomal chromosomae were discovered, making the chrosomal count forty-eight.

Contrary to this Ford[28] has reported finding only 46 chromosomes instead of the expected 47 in bone marrow calls of a mongol girl. This child was selected for examination for the mother was only 21 years old when the child was born. Although there is at present an extensive literature concerning the origin of chromosome structural changes, also spoken of as chromosome rearrangements or chromosome aberrations, I quite agree with Ford, who states: "Doubtless the next few years will bring a big increase in our knowledge of the types of chromosomal abnormality to which mankind is subject, and estimates of the frequencies with which they occur. These frequencies, like those of many other characteristics, may be found to differ somewhat between different ethnic groups. All of this will be valuable information in its own right."

SUMMARY

Up to the present writing three groups of persons with abnormal chromosome numbers have been described: (1) mongols[8] with 47 chromosomes, the extra one being a small arocentric autosome; (2) persons[23] with the chromatin-positive form of Klinefelter's syndrome, with 47 chromosomes and a sex formula XXY; and (3) females[10, 11] with Turner's syndrome who are chromatin-negative, with 45 chromosomes and a chromosomal sex formula XO. It is postulated that the XO and XXY configurations arise from non-disjunction when reduction divisions should have occurred during miosis. Gordon[24] believes that a girl with chromatin-negative Turner's syndrome has an XO configuration, and not XY, and therefore should not be described as having a "male chromatin pattern." "Similarly," states Gordon, "the man with chromatin-positive Klinefelter's syndrome should not be traumatized with the news that he has 'a female chromatin pattern.' " (4) Another type of sex chromosome anomaly has been reported. This is the so-called "super-female type." Jacobs *et al.*,[26] report such a female characterized by a chromosome number of 47 and a chromosome sex formula XXX. In appraising this form of chromosome anomaly, Gordon rightly objects to the term "super-female" and recommends terms as B.B., DD or MM.

REFERENCES

1. Ford, C. E.: *Human Chromosomes.* In Symposium on Nuclear Sex, edited by Smith, D. R., and Davidson, W. M. Inter Science Publishers, Inc., New York, p. 13-19, 1958.
2. Klinger, H. P.: The sex chromatin body. Its finer structure and behavior during amitosis or endomitosis. In Symposium on *Nuclear Sex,* edited by Smith, D. R., and Davidson, W. M. Inter Science Publishers, Inc., New York, p. 20-23, 1958.
3. Sachs, L., and Danon, M.: The genetic implications of nuclear sexing. In Symposium on *Nuclear Sex,* edited by Smith, D. R., and Davidson, W. M. Inter Science Publishers, Inc., New York, p. 42-45, 1958.

4. Danon, M., and Sachs, L.: The sex chromosomes and the development of human intersexes. In Symposium on *Nuclear Sex*, edited by Smith, D. R., and Davidson, W. M. Inter Science Publishers, Inc., New York, p. 55-61, 1958.
5. Ford, C. E., and Hamerton, J. L.: Chromosomes of man. *Nature, London, 178:* 1020-1023, 1956.
6. Tjio, J. H., and Levan, A.: Chromosome number of man. *Hereditas, 42:* 1-6, 1956.
7. Ford, C. E.: Human cytogenetics; its present place and future possibilities. *Am. J. Human Genet., 12:* 104-117, 1960.
8. LeJeune, J., Gautier, M., and Turpin, R.: Études des chromosomes somatiques de neuf enfants mongoliens. *Compt. rend. Acad. d. Sc., 248:* 1721, 1959.
9. Jacobs, P. A., and Strong, J. A.: Case of human intersexuality having possible XXY sex-determining mechanism. *Nature, London, 183:* 302, 1959.
10. Ford, C. E., Jones, K. W., Polani, P. E., de Almeida, J. C., and Briggs, J. H.: Sex-chromosome anomaly in case of gonadal dysgenesis (Turner's Syndrome). *Lancet, 1:* 711-713, 1959.
11. Fraccaro, M., Kaijser, K., and Lindsten, J.: Chromosome complement in gonadal dysgenesis (Turner's Syndrome). *Lancet, 1:* 886, 1959.
12. Jacobs, P. A., et al.: Evidence for existence of human "super female." *Lancet, 2:* 423-425, 1959.
13. Bar, M., and Bertram, E. G.: A morphological distinction between the neurons of the male and female and its behavior of the nucleolar satellites. *Nature, 163:* 676, 1949.
14. Barr, M., and Murray, L.: Sex chromatin and phenotype in man. *Science, 130:* 679-685, Sept., 1959.
15. Lennox, B., Serr, D. M., and Ferguson-Smith, M. A.: The sex chromatin in Memoirs of the Society for Endocrinology No. 7, *Sex Differentiation and Development.* University Press, Cambridge, 1960.
16. Moore, K. L., and Barr, M.: Nuclear morphology according to sex in human tissues. *Acta. Anat., 21:* 197, 1954.
17. Yerganian, G.: Duality of the mammalian X-chromosome and its genetic implications. Presented at the meeting of the American Society of Human Genetics, Memphis, Tennessee, April, 1960.
18. Stanbury, J. B.: In discussion of case presentation No. 46341, Case Records of the Massachusetts General Hospital. *New England J. Med., 263:* 401, 1960.
19. Marberger, E., Boccabella, R. A., and Nelson, W. O.: Oral smear as a method of chromosomal sex detection. *Proc. Soc. Exper. Biol. & Med., 89:* 488, 1955.
20. Guard, H. R.: A new technique for differential staining of the sex chromatin, and the determination of its incidence in exfoliated vaginal epithelial cells. *Am. J. Clin. Path., 32:* 145, Aug., 1959.

21. Davidson, W. M., and Smith, D. R.: A morphological sex difference in the polymorphonuclear neutrophil leucocytes. *Brit. M. J., 2:* 6, 1954.
22. Lennox, B., Serr, D. M., and Ferguson-Smith, M. A.: The sex chromatin in Memoirs of the Society for Endocrinology No. 7, *Sex Differentiation and Development.* University Press, Cambridge, 1960.
23. Ford, C. E., Polani, P. E., Briggs, J. H., and Bishop, P. M. F.: Presumptive human XXY/XX. Mosaic. *Nature, London, 183:* 1030-1032, April 11, 1959.
24. Gordon, G. S.: *The Reproductive System.* Year Book Publishers, Inc., Chicago, p. 297, 1959-1960 Series.
25. Moore, K. L., Graham, M. A., and Bakr, M. L.: The detection of chromosomal sex in hermaphrodites from a skin biopsy. *Surg. Gynec. & Obst., 96:* 641, 1953.
26. Jacobs, P. A., Baikie, A. G., Courtbrown, W. M., and Strong, J. A.: The somatic chromosomes in mongolism. *Lancet, 1:* 710, 1959.
27. Ford, C. E., Jones, K. W., Miller, O. J., Mittwoch, V., Penrose, L. S., Ridler, M., Shapiro, A.: The chromosomes in a patient showing both mongolism and the Klinefelter's syndrome. *Lancet, 1:* 709, 1959.
28. Ford, C. E.: *Chromosomal Abnormality and Congenital Malformation in Ciba Foundation Symposium on Congenital Malformations.* Editors: Wolstenholme, W. E. G., and O'Connor, M. C. Little, Brown and Co., Boston, 1960.

Chapter 7

SEX AND ITS DETERMINATIONS

THE PRESENCE of the testes has always been an important index to sex and its assignment. Indeed it has been traditional since the onset of time for the accoucher to carefully examine the newborn infant and determine whether the mother has delivered a boy or girl. The decision[1, 2, 3, 4, 5, 6, 7, 8] may not always be simple and accurate. It is estimated that undifferentiated external genitalia at birth occurs in one of every thousand babies.[6] With the birth of a pseudo-hermaphrodite, one cannot tell from the *appearance of the external genitalia* just what is the sex of the new born child. Fortunately many tests are now available which may serve as an aid in determining the true sex of the new born. In the previous chapters, these various tests have been described and clinically applied. In this section these tests will be applied to the determination of sex, assignment of sex and re-assignment of sex.

In all cases of questionable doubt as to the sex of the infant, the chromatin nuclear test is the first test that should be utilized. If the test proves to be positive, and on a basis of incidence above, it would be safe to assume that the confusion regarding the correct sex is due to adrenal hyperplasia. It might also be the result of non-adrenal pseudohermaphroditism (less common) or may actually be a case of true hermaphroditism (extremely rare).

The investigation must now turn to evaluation of 17-ketosteroids (see Chapter 5). If the assay reveals that the 17-ketosteroids are markedly elevated and the child is chromatin positive one can assume that the underlying cause is definitely due to congenital adrenal hyperplasia resulting in pseudo-hermaphroditism in the female (macrogenitosomia praecox in the male). As previously stated,[10] such a disturbance is the direct result of hypersecretion of the adrenal cortex. This may be due to hyperplasia or more rarely with tumor of the adrenal cortex. At birth confusion in the determination of sex is created because of markedly enlarged clitoris with malformation of the external genitalia. Thus female pseudo-hermaphroditism is suspected purely on the clinical picture and confirmed by the findings of elevated urinary 17-ketosteroids.

The question often arises as to whether the determination of urinary 17-ketosteroids might be equivocal. In such cases the test should be repeated in several weeks. Others[11,12] recommend the determination of pregnanetriol, for the most recent developments seem to confirm that pregnanetriolone is said to occupy 65% of this steroid fraction. This is most diagnostic of congenital adrenal hyperplasia.[13] In cases of continued doubt, the reader should be reminded, that patients with bilateral hyperplasia can be inhibited in their production of ACTH by the administration of cortisone, to such an extent that there will be a definite drop in the amount of 17-ketosteroids or of the pregnanetriol excreted in the urine.* In the presence of adrenocortical tumor there is no significant decrease in the production of urinary 17-ketosteroids despite the administration of cortisone.

The reader should also bear in mind that these children with an enlarged clitoris may be confused with a small penis, and the child accepted as a male and erroneously brought up as a male. The hypertrophied clitoris closely resembles a hypospadic penis bound ventrally in a position of chordee with marked variations in the degree of fusion of the labioscrotal folds. No gonads are palpable within the fused scrotal folds which often has given the physician the erroneous impression of male cryptorchidism, when in reality the child is a female pseudohermaphrodite.[3] Urethroscopic examination of the urogenital sinus in questionable cases will reveal the communication with the vagina and the cervix of the uterus can often be visualized.

As previously stated the adreno-genital syndrome is more prevalent among females[4,14,15] but there is a form of congenital adrenal hyperplasia in males (chromatin negative) spoken of as macrogenitosomia praecox. It is analogous to pseudo-hermaphroditism

---

*See footnote, Chapter 5.

found in females except that genital development is *isosexual.* In this condition there is no confusion regarding the *determination of sex* but there is alarm as to the sexual precocity. The penis grows to adult proportions at any early age. In some cases the child may reach the age of three without any unusual genital manifestations. Sexual development is usually rapid and sexual hair and acne develop early. *Although the genitalia are of adult size, the testes remain small and immature* and spermatogenesis does not occur.

It follows from the above outline that variations in the appearance of the genitalia may lead to confusion as to the determination and assignment of sex.[5,16,17] Such confusion unfortunately can lead to erroneous assignment of sex. When this occurs much uncertainty and despair may be associated with the ultimate raising and development of the child. Whenever there is any doubt about the child's sex, accepted tests should be utilized as soon as possible. Should the tests be questionable they should be repeated within five to six weeks, and during this period of time no absolute declaration of sex be made. I quite agree with Hampson[18] who states: "It is far better to leave the parents in a state of uncertainty during this interval than to make a temporary declaration of sex and cause the parents to go through the ordeal of changing the information that has got around ··· It is not easy for any parent to face telling well-wishing friends and neighbors that the doctors are not sure what the baby is, but in the long run it is vastly preferable that they say this than to go back when the baby is four or five weeks old and say, 'the doctors have changed their minds.' "

The final assignment of sex in any given person can only be made after careful evaluation of all available data. No relative values can be assigned. All factors are important and serve to give a definite architectural pattern which should help in making the proper assignment of sex. Thus the assignment of sex should be one that fits (a) chromosal sex; (b) gonadal sex; (c) morphology of external genitalia; (d) status of internal genitalia; (e) hormonal sex; (f) sex of rearing; and (g) gender sex.

(a) Chromosomal Sex

Knowledge of chromosomal sex is of great aid if there is doubt about a person's sex. It is of significant value since clinically it can be utilized quickly and accurately. Our present concept of the chromosomal pattern of the individual's cells is as follows: The sex chromosome in the male is made up of an X and Y element while the female sex chromosome is made up of two X elements. When the sex chromosome divided during maturation, each ovum, therefore carries an X element while half the sperm carry an X and half carry a Y element. Thus depending upon what kind of sperm unites with the ovum at fertilization, the resulting individual carries an XX or XY sex chromosome in each of its cells. This classic concept of sex formerly envisioned the union of X and Y chromosome as sex determining of the gonad and today is accepted as also influencing the fate of the Wolffian and Müllerian ducts and the morphology of the external genitalia.

This advancement in idea differs from the former belief that the gonad was the definite arbiter and final determinant of sex. The belief that the individual's clinical sex always corresponded to the chromosomal sex, has now been questioned by patients with gonadal dysgenesis, formerly called ovarian agenesis or Turner's syndrome, who were considered to be female, have now been found in most cases to have the XY chromosome pattern. Equally contradictory is that patients with testicular hypoplasia (Klinefelter's syndrome), have male characteristics, but in some cases have a female XX chromosome pattern. Nevertheless evaluations of nuclear sex cannot be denied as an important aid in the determination of sex.

(b) Gonadal Sex

Kleb's[19] well-known classification of hermaphrodites is the identification of the sex of the gonads by microscopic examination. The Kleb's classification as originally proposed is impractical today for at times other criteria of sex contradict the gonadal sex. It must be remembered that the primitive gonad is indeterminate, and during development there are periods in which the gonadal pattern of first one sex and then the other is predominant. Further the conversion of a gonad of one type to that of another type is not impossible. Successful therapy is often dependent upon gonadal sex determination and this should be determined by microscopic examination since the gross appearance of gonads in cases of suspected intersexuality may be entirely misleading.

(c) Status of External Genitalia

The assignment of sex to a new-born is universally determined by the status and appearance of the external genitalia. Thus the sexual assignment and the sexual rearing of most persons has been the result of the obstetrician's decision at child-birth. Where the assignment has been erroneously made because of vague anatomical differentiation, the patient often, but not always, became acclimated to the role determined by the assignment and sexual rearing.

Here the general rule to follow is: individuals with ambiguity of sexing should be assigned a practical sex before gender role exerts its influence (see gender role). The use of the chromosomal test in such cases is of value but not entirely without error. For example the chromosomal test does not differentiate true from pseudo-hermaphroditism although it definitely provides ancillary data. When a baby has gonads in the scrotum or in the groins, but is chromatin positive, Klinefelter's syndrome or true hermaphroditis may be suspected. But, if the child presents gynecoid genitals and is chromatin negative, male pseudohermaphroditism should be suspected and Klinefelter's syndrome can be ruled out.

Hamblen[6] suggests that when the external genitalia appear audroid and the child is chromatin positive, female pseudohermaphroditism due to congenital adrenal hyperplasia should be the tentative diagnosis until diagnostic studies eliminate this possibility. As stated above, elevation of 17-ketosteroids is of great diagnostic value and when such tests are ambiguous, the demonstration of pregnanetriol in the urine will confirm the diagnosis of adrenal hyperplasia.

The assignment of sex to a new-born cannot always be effectively determined by the appearance and status of the external genitalia. This is well demonstrated by the following case:

A four year old boy was admitted to the hospital because his parents were concerned about a definite lowering of the child's voice which at first had been mistaken for a cold. He had grown rapidly in the past 4 months and acne had developed. Upon examination of the genitalia, one was impressed with the large phallus and the comparatively small testes. Hypospadias was present, and marked coarse hair was seen in the pubic region. The chromatin test was positive but urethroscopy failed to reveal a vagina or cervix. Exploratory laparotomy revealed a normal uterus, normal ovaries and fallopian tubes.*

(d) Status of the Internal Genitalia

In the section devoted to normal embryology, emphasis was placed upon the accepted theory that in every normal embryo both the Wolffian and Müllerian ducts are present and capable of development into internal male or internal female genitalia. The *differentiation is made by the hormone of environment.* When, as a result of some disturbance in the normal progress of development, an anatomical alteration may occur and the internal genitalia may then develop in a contradictory fashion. Under such circumstances the determination of such contradiction is essential for proper sex status.[7]

The status of the internal genitalia can only be determined by exploratory laparotomy, as in the case just described, and although it is not necessarily a prerequisite to sex assignment it cannot be denied that when performed all sexual ambiguities will receive the proper assignment. I do not believe corrective surgery should be performed within the first few days of life. I do believe that exploration is indicated and will save many anxious days if not years on the part of the parents, who can then definitely be told what sex or what preponderant sex (taking into consideration all anatomical factors) should be elected and planned for future habilitation.

(e) Hormonal Sex

The so-called secondary sex characteristics such as body structure, breast development, hair growth, fat distribution, general

---

*In contrast see case report on p. 78.

body habitus, are all important as a criterion of sex. These factors play an important role in the proper understanding of cases of intersex.

(f) Sex of Rearing

The role of the assigned sex and the rearing of such assignment is of singular importance. Such an individual's assignment must be one that will be accepted by society. Jones[8] and Scott believe that of the various criteria of sex, the sex of rearing is the most obvious and one that can be recognized by the community as well as by the physician. Sexual behavior and orientation as a man or woman can be greatly influenced by the rearing inaugurated after sex assignment at birth. Here, too, careful consideration of these influencing factors must be made in all clinical cases of intersex.

(g) Gender Sex

This is the greater role played by the individual. It is an important phychological criterion of sex and often one of the key notes in sex assignment, particularly in early cases where questionable sex assignment is an issue. This is determined by personality study of the patient in which his actions, mannerisms, speech, likes and dislikes are carefully evaluated. For example does the patient like football or sewing; fishing and not cooking? Is the patient more assertative as a well behaved boy or more retiring as a well behaved girl? Other personality traits must be scrutinized. According to Hampson,[18] gender role is not something that is automatically or instinctively determined. It is, "All things that a person does or says to disclose himself or herself as having the status of a man or boy or of a girl or woman,··· it is something that is cumulatively built up during the course of all the experiences and transactions of growing up··· It includes, for instance, dress, name, haircut, fantasies, posture, gesture, mannerisms, affections, daydreams, ambitions for the future. It includes all these things, and more besides."

Although the psychologic study of very young children is by no means easy, such investigation has revealed a great deal of valuable information. Money[7] and the Hampsons have studied a large group of such individuals and believe that "gender role" becomes fixed at an early age and for this reason do not advocate change of assigned sex except at a very early age. At a recent panel discussion, Hampson[1] stated: "We feel that the infant at birth is quite undifferentiated in terms of having a specific gender role. We feel further, that during the early years of childhood, gender role is cumulatively built up. The age by which a person's gender role is fairly definitely established seems to vary. By and large, the child does not seem to have established a very firm and inflexible gender role or sense of being a boy, or sense of being a girl, before the age of 18 months or two years. We feel further therefore, that it is reasonable from the psychologic point of view to make reassignment of sex up to a year or 18 months··· There might be other instances where, at four years, a child's gender role was not completely fixed, and where there may be a reasonable possibility that a person could establish himself in the opposite gender role if all other factors pointed to a change as being a tremendous advantage to the child."

REASSIGNMENT OF SEX

Wilkens,[3,4,5] who has had great experience in sex differentiation in children, states: "In the past, serious abnormalities of sex differentiation have often remained unsuspected until puberty. Frequently, the ambiguity of the genitalia has confused the physician so that he has refrained from making any decision until secondary sexual characteristics develop. The parents have been left in anxiety and doubt with a 'half-boy and half-girl.' At times, the child has been changed back and forth from one sex to another. He grows up in a state of uncertainty and confusion and at puberty may be subjected to a startling surprise ··· With recent advantages of knowledge, it is now possible within the first few months of life to make a firm and rational decision in regard to the appropriate sex of rearing and to start or plan any corrective procedures."

Reassignment of sex often becomes necessary and, when it does, factors of religion as well as legal problems arise. Such reassignment may occur because the physician ultimately finds that the initially assigned sex is not a practical one. At other times reassignment is requested because of pressure from the parents. At other times, the patient requests reassignment.

Sex reassignment is best performed before 24 months of age, for the gender role at this time has not as yet been established. However some workers believe it occurs earlier (18 months). When the reassignment is performed after the establishment of gender role serious psychological problems are encountered and change of sex by edict is not recommended.

Burns *et al.*,[20] in writing on reassignment of sex, report three cases of reassignment of sex, representing three different clinical entities. The first case was a male with third degree hypospadias, erroneously considered to be a female at birth. While working as a nurse's aid in a female medical ward, attention of the medical staff was aroused by the necessity of daily shaving, the presence of superfluous hair on the arms, a male type of larynx with a moderately pitched voice and no evidence of female breasts. The patient was anxious for therapy and stated "he" had always remained largely to himself, but was emotionally attracted to females, having several times attempted sexual intercourse with females. This has always been unsuccessful because of a pronounced ventral curvature of the phallus, made worse with erection. When examined a mid-scrotal type of hypospadias was noted, with a well developed normal-looking scrotum with a normal testicle on the left side and no testicle on the right side. "He" had previously had an appendectomy, at which time an unidentified mass was removed. Digital rectal examination revealed a normal prostate with normal prostatic secretion. Panendoscopy revealed normal male prostatic urethra with a rudimentary verumontanum. Exploratory revealed no internal female genitalia and no testicle could be found on the right side. Hypospadic repair was performed and *the sex reassigned to male.*

"The patient's psychologic readjustment has been most satisfactory. He is now in the eleventh postoperative year and has been married for 3½ years. Premarital sterility studies showed no evidence of sperm. Both he and his wife report highly satisfactory sexual function and profess to be extremely happy."

The second case was that of a female pseudo-hermaphrodite with congenital adrenocortical hyperplasia, as confirmed by elevated 17-ketosteroid excretion, which could be depressed by cortisone therapy; pan-endoscopy revealed a normal female type of urethra; absent prostate on digital rectal examination; visualization of normal cervix and vagina. Exploration revealed a normal uterus, fallopian tubes and ovaries. Cortisone therapy was continued and clitoris subsequently amputated. Burns[20] states: "A point of considerable interest in this case was that in spite of the fact that this child had been reared as a male for 4 years, a male gender role never actually developed. The child had always ben interested in dolls and dresses and was never attracted to trucks and trains and other toys that ordinarily interest male children."

In the third case, no opinion regarding gender pattern could be formulated by the authors. In view of a strongly positive chromatin sex pattern and normal internal female genitalia it was believed that such a child's development would most likely follow a female pattern and be adaptable to normal female environment. The phallus was amputated and plastic reconstruction of the existing vaginal orifice performed.

On the other hand there are those who believe that individuals living with an hermaphrodite contradiction, uncorrected for many years should not be denied correction, i.e., correction of sex. Such adults, usually in early adult life, are cognizant or suspicious of some mistake having been made and serious consideration should be given to such cases. In fact such persons who suspect a mistake and request a change of sex have actually reassigned themselves. This is borne out in many clinical cases, and is well illustrated in the following case reported by Albert:[1]

"A girl was born with ambiguous external genitalia. The family doctor said the baby was a girl. Hence the baby was raised as a girl. At puberty she became masculinized and began to have masculine interests. She persisted in her feminine role simply to please her parents. There was no psychiatric evaluation at all. However, the conflict between the girl and her parents grew. On the one hand she did not want to displease her parents who insisted that she be feminine. On the other hand she felt masculine. She resolved the conflict simply by leaving home and going to California. On the way she obtained a boy's haircut and boy's clothes. She then got a job in an airplane factory as a male. Later 'she' fell in love with a girl, lived with her a while, decided that this was 'her' way of life, and appeared wanting to be transformed physically as completely as possible into a male. The hypospadias was corrected. 'She' married her girl and lived happily as a married man having intercourse two or three times a day and urinating as a male."

Albert in discussing this case states: "We will not argue that this individual did or did not have serious doubts as to her sex all along. There is no psychiatric documentation that after she reassigned herself, she was psychologically healthy or unhealthy. We have only her statement that she was a happily married man, and functionally so at least in the two respects mentioned. Thus, this sex reassignment represented a fait accomplished as far as we are concerned. Such individuals do not go to psychiatrists to find out about their imprinting. They have made up their minds and appear before a urologist requesting appropriate measures."

A word about masculinization of female fetus due to use of orally given progestins administered to mothers as treatment of habitual or threatened abortion.*[22,23,24,25,26] As stated above female pseudo-hermaphroditism due to congenital adrenal hyperplasia is an accepted clinical condition. Embryonic masculinization of the external genitalia has been reported by various authors following the administration of 17-a-ethinylestosterone and other similar steroids. In many cases a markedly masculinized female infant is readily mistaken for a hypospadic male or a normal male with simple cryptorchism. These infants differ from patients with adreno-genital syndrome due to cortical hyperplasia (or tumor) in that they do not have elevated levels of urinary 17-ketosteroids. With growth they do not show progressive virilization with precocious growth of pubic hair or accelerated growth and accelerated osseous development.[27,28,29] Indeed as emphasized by Wilkins,[24] these patients at puberty exhibit normal feminization, with menstruation and ovulation.

---

*See summary at end of Chapter 2 (Embryonic Gonadal Differentiation).

It is believed by many that non-adrenal female pseudo-hermaphrodites should always be raised as girls. The parents should be reassured that the child will develop as a normal girl and mature into a normal, fertile woman. Hormonal therapy is not recommended in these cases.

If at birth the appearance of the child is suggestive of female pseudohermaphroditism, buccal smear tests should be performed at once. This will reveal "chromatin-positive" type of nuclei. In addition one will find normal levels of urinary 17-ketosteroids.* When a urogenital sinus further complicates the picture, it is advisable to have a urethroscopic examination to demonstrate the communicating vagina and cervix. It may be necessary (in rare cases) to exclude the possibility of true hermaphroditism with both testes and ovaries. This can best be accomplished by exploratory laparotomy, which will also confirm the status of the internal genitalia.

The doctor faced with a problem of sex assignment is indeed confronted with a serious task. To make the decision at an early age is even a greater responsibility and I strongly oppose those who in a "god-like manner" believe they are capable of making such decisions. These problems are well demonstrated in the following two cases:

> D. H., a three and one half year old negro male was re-admitted to the urological service of the Metropolitan Hospital for sex determination. He had been born in this hospital and at the time of his birth it was noted that he had the following malformations of his external genitalia. He had a perineal hypospadias; labia-like cleft scrotum and bilateral palpable gonads in the groin. Cystoscopy, intravenous pyelograms, and cystogram at this time were accepted as within normal range.

---

*The reader is referred to chapter 5, describing the 17-ketosteroids but for sake of continuity of the pertinent data it is here repeated: The nature of the adrenal pathology will determine the level of the urinary 17-ketosteroids. High urinary excretion values of the 17-ketosteroids are seen in malignant tumor of the adrenal cortex but this is rarely seen in children or in infants. In adults with virilism without demonstrable adrenal cortex pathology, the urinary neutral 17-ketosteroids are usually normal or only slightly increased. Virilism present in a child before puberty will usually demonstrate elevated neutral urinary 17-ketosteroids.

At present admission, he has a normal size phallus for age 3½. There is no demonstrable penile urethra but a definite perineal opening not more than 1 cm. in depth which contains the urethra. The scrotum is not developed and is cleft-like, resembling labia folds, within which the gonads could be palpated. Laboratory work was entirely within normal limits for the initial evaluation of 17-ketosteroids which were 3.8 mg. for a 55 cc specimen. Intravenous pyelograms and cystogram were again described as being within normal limits. Cystoscopy revealed no evidence of verumontanum or prostatic urethra. Exploratory laparotomy was performed. No female organs or vestigial remnants of female organs were demonstrated. The palpable gonads were exposed and identified as testicles with normal epididymes. Bilateral testicular biopsies were taken and reported as normal testes in keeping with the patient's age. Buccal smear reported as male positive. At the weekly urological conference controversial opinions were raised as to therapy and question of reassignment of sex. It was felt by the majority of the staff that we were dealing with a case of perineal hypospadias, cryptorchidism and micropenis. Hormone therapy was instigated and the child is to be kept under observation.

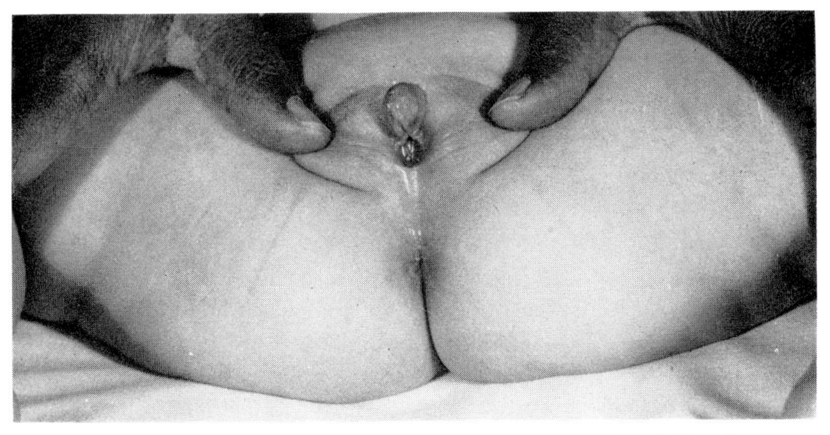

Fig. 11. Photograph of external genitalia of 3½ year old child whose sex was in doubt. The gonads were palpable in the lateral folds. Photomicrograph of biopsy of testes are demonstrated in Figure 2. Laparotomy revealed no female organs. This is a case of perineal hypospadias, cryptorchidism and micro-penis.

At about the same time, S. S., a child age 5, was admitted to the urological service with a chief complaint of "two sexes." The child was born at another hospital and at the time of birth, the sex was not definitely assigned. The mother stated that during her pregnancy she attended the out-patient department and was treated extensively with injections and some green-brown capsules, but did not know the nature of the oral medication or intra-muscular injections. She had constant nausea, vomiting and abdominal pains throughout the pregnancy. Delivery was uneventful. Patient is the first child to the mother. A three year old brother is normal. Previous hospital records were obtained and summary is as follows:

> Patient was first seen at the age of seven weeks. Physical examination revealed very short phallus with meatus at tip of phallus. Gonads were palpable in the scrotum or what looked like fused labia majora. No female organs were palpable on rectal examination. At this time the impression was that of a male pseudo-hermaphrodite. One month later buccal smear was done and again reported as chromatin negative. Skin biopsy was taken from thigh and this was reported as showing male chromatin pattern. Urethrograms were attempted but were unsatisfactory due to scanty filling (non-diagnostic). Two months later examination again showed meatus to be at tip of penis, and three months later phallus measured 1.5 cm long and 0.5 cm wide. Testes were normal.
>
> Five years later, child now (see Fig. 12) demonstrates a small phallus in normal position. It is slightly enlarged for a clitoris and very small (1½ cm) for a normal penis (micropenis). The glans is not characteristic and is partially covered by a short prepuce. There is a hypospadic urethral meatus placed in the base of this small phallus. The rest of the urethra can be palpated through the scrotum. There is a scrotum with a median raphe but without any characteristic rugae. Within, 2 hemiscrotum gonads are palpable, and appear to be testes because epididymus structure can be identified on manual palpation. The perineal urethra could be palpated normally. Rectal palpation revealed a small prostate and no evidence of uterus or broad ligament. Cystoscopy

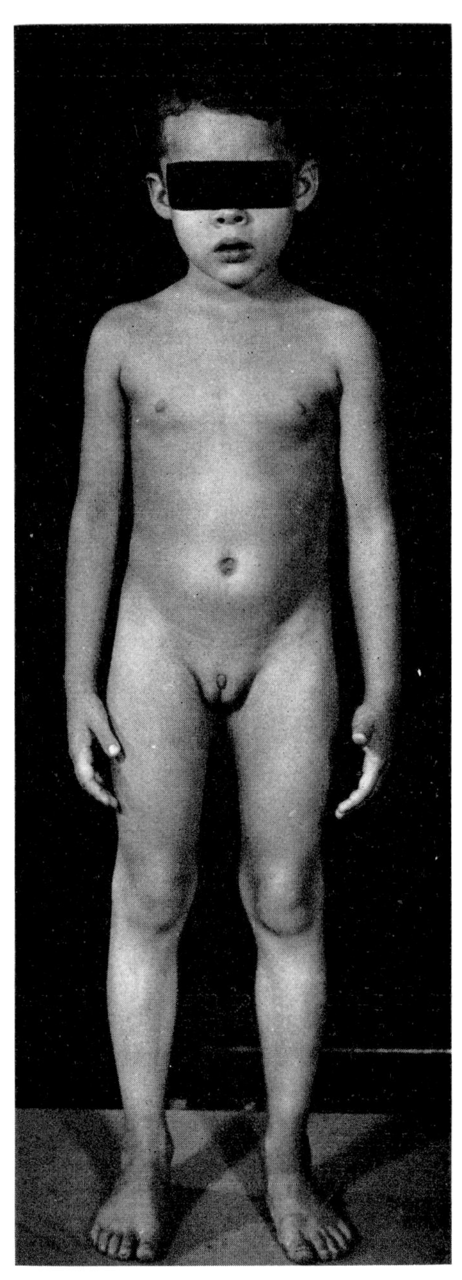

FIG. 12. Photograph of 5 year old child originally diagnosed as male-pseudohermaphrodite. Male chromatin pattern on repeated skin and buccal mucosa. Small phallus in normal position, palpable gonads in scrotum with median raphe but without characteristic rugae. Hypospadic urethral meatus at base of penis. Cystoscopy revealed small veru montanum in normal location.

showed normal bladder mucosa and both right and left ureteral meati could be identified. A small veru montanum was identified in normal location.

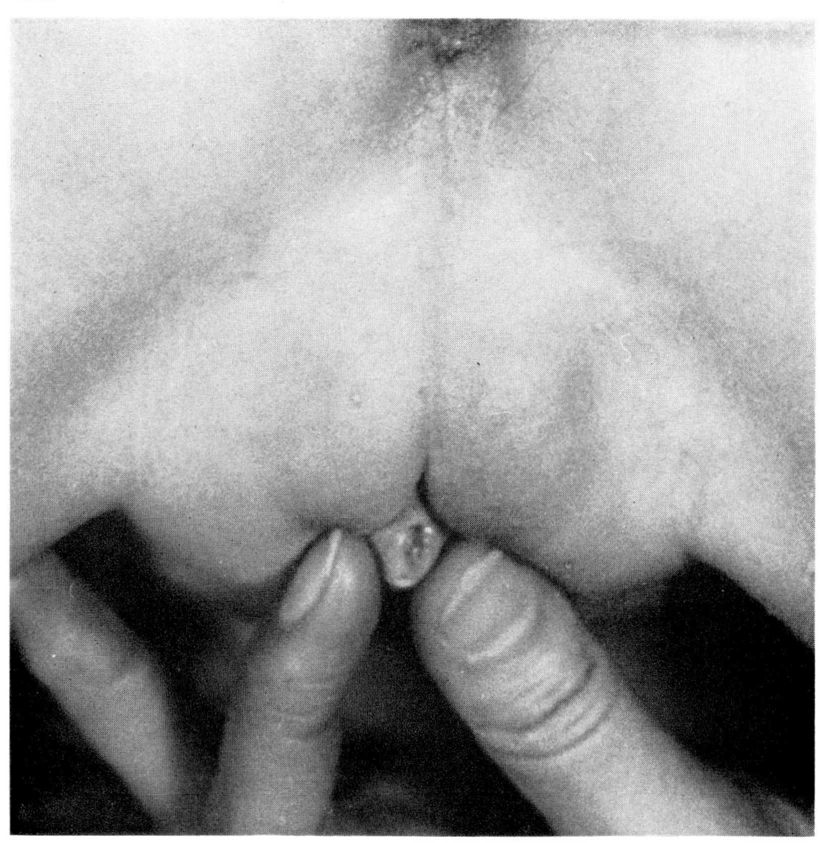

FIG. 13. Close up of photograph of genitalia of 5 year old child demonstrated in Figure 12.

All[3] are agreed that a diagnosis of male pseudohermaphroditism can be made with certainty in a child with genitalia of equivocal sexuality, providing both testicles are palpable, verumontanum is demonstrated on endoscopy, sex chromatin is of a male pattern, and 17-ketosteroids urinary excretion is not elevated. In all cases the management depends entirely upon the circumstances in which the child is brought up. When the child is recognized as a male, development is uncomplicated but when he is put in the female category many complications ensue, which often results in a reassignment of sex in later life. Unfortunately too many cases of hypospadias of a severe degree have been classified as cases of male pseudohermaphroditism, requiring sex assignment to the opposite sex.

Just because a male is born with incomplete masculine development of the external genitalia, is no reason for reassigning his sex to that of a female, unless he possesses purely feminine external genitalia. Many[3,4,6,7] pediatricians and endocrinologists believe that in males unless the phallus is well developed the patient cannot function as a male and will be subjected to constant humiliation and embarassment throughout life and should therefore be reared as a female. The author does not accept this broad statement and as stated previously would recommend reassignment of sex only in those males with female external genitalia. Such males usually feminize at puberty under the influence of estrogen secreted by the testes and often marry and lead normal lives despite the fact that they do not menstruate and are obviously sterile.

REFERENCES

1. Bunge, R., Moderator; Albert, A., Burns, E., and Hampson, J., Collaborators. Panel Discussion: Determination of sex and what to do about it. *J. Urol.*, Vol. 81, No. 1, Jan. 1959.
2. Steiner, M. M.: Modern concepts of urologic endocrinology. *J. Urol.*, Vol. 81, No. 1, Jan., 1959.
3. Wilkins, L.: *Diagnosis and Treatment of Endocrine Disorders in Childhood and Adolescence,* Ed. 2. Thomas, Springfield, 1957.
4. Wilkins, L.: Abnormalities and variations of sexual development during childhood and adolescence. *Advances in Pediat., 3:* 159, 1948.
5. Wilkins, L., Grumbach, M. M., Van Wyk, J. J., Shephard, T. H., and Papadatos, C.: Hermaphroditism; Classification, Diagnosis, Selection of Sex and Treatment. *Pediatrics, 16:* 303, 1955.
6. Hamblen, E. C.: The assignment of sex to an individual; some enigmas and some practical clinical criteria. *Am. J. Obst. and Gynec.,* 74: 1228-1244, 1957.
7. Money, J., Hampson, J. G., and Hampson, J. L.: Hermaphroditism; recommendations concerning assignment of sex, change of sex and psychologic management. *Bull. Johns Hopkins Hospital, 97:* 284, 1955.

8. Jones, H. W., Jr., and Scott, W. W.: *Hermaphroditism, Genital Anomalies and Related Endocrine Disorders.* Williams and Wilkins Co., Baltimore, 1958.
9. Moore, K. L., and Barr, M. L.: Nuclear morphology according to sex, in human tissue. *Acta Anat., 21:* 197, 1954.
10. Sohval, A.: Diseases of the Testis. In Soffer: *Diseases of the Endocrine Glands.* Lea and Febiger, 1958.
11. Fisher, A. H., and Riley, C. L.: Pregnanediol excretion in a masculinizing syndrome. *J. Clin. Endocrin. & Med., 12:* 891, 1952.
12. Bongiovanni, A. M.: The detection of pregnandiol and pregnantriol in the urine of patients with adrenal hyperplasia. Suppression with cortisone; preliminary report. *Bull. Johns Hopkins Hospital, 92:* 244, 1953.
13. Mason, H. L., and Kepler, E. J.: Isolation of steroids from urine of patients with adrenal cortical tumors and adrenal hyperplasia; new 17-ketosteroids, and andosterone-3, 11-diol-17-one. *J. Biol. Chem., 161:* 235, 1945.
14. Goldstein, E. A., Rubin, S. W., and Askin, J. A.: Carcinoma of adrenal cortex with adrenogenital syndrome in children. *Am. J. Dis. Child., 72:* 563, 1946.
15. Melicow, M. M., and Cahill, G. F.: The role of the adrenal cortex in somato-sexual disturbances in infants and children; A clinico-pathologic analysis. *J. Clin. Endocrin., 10:* 24, 1950.
16. Gross, R. E., and Meeker, I. A.: Abnormalities of sexual development. *Pediatrics, 16:* 303, 1955.
17. Money, J.: Hermaphroditism quoted by Wilkins, Grumbach, Van Wyk, Shephard, Papadatos. Unpublished doctoral thesis. Harvard University Library, 1952.
18. Hampson, J.: In Panel Discussion: Determination of sex and what to do about it. *J. Urol.* Vol. 81, No. 1, Jan. 1959.
19. Klebs, E.: *Handbuch der pathologisch en anatomie.* August Hirchwald, Berlin, 1876.
20. Burns, E., Segaloff, A., and Carrera, G. M.: Reassignment of sex; Report of 3 cases. *J. Urol., 84:* 126, 1960.
21. Young, H. H.: *Congenital Abnormalities, Hermaphroditism and Related Adrenal Diseases.* The Williams and Wilkins Co., Baltimore, 1937.
22. Wilkins, L.: A feminizing adrenal tumor causing gynecomastia in a boy of five years contrasted with a viriling tumor in a five year old girl. *J. Clin. Endocrinol., 8:* 111, Feb., 1948.
23. Wilkins, L.: *Diagnosis and Treatment of Endocrine Disorders in Childhood and Adolescence.* Ed. 2, Thomas, Springfield, 1957.
24. Wilkins, L.: Masculinization of female fetus due to use of orally given progestins. *J.A.M.A., 172:* 1028-1032, 1960.

25. Wilkins, L., Jones, H. W., Holman, G. H., and Stempfel, R. S., Jr.: Masculinization of the female fetus associated with administration of oral and intramuscular progestins during gestation; Non-adrenal female pseudo-hermaphroditism. *J. Clin. Endocrinol. & Metab., 18:* 559-585, 1958.
26. Wilkins, L.: Masculinization of the female fetus due to use of certain synthetic oral progestins during pregnancy. *Arch. Anat. Microscop. et Morphol. Explt., 48:* (supp.) 313-329, 1959.
27. Grumbach, M. M., Ducharme, J. R., and Moloshok, R. E.: On the fetal masculinizing action of certain oral progestins. *J. Clin. Endocrinol., 19:* 1369, 1959.
28. Grumbach, M. M., and Ducharme, J. R.: The effects of androgens on fetal sexual development. *J. Fertility and Sterility, 11:* 157, 1960.
29. Jones, H. W., and Wilkins, L.: The genital anomaly associated with prenatal exposure to progestogens. *J. Fertility and Sterility, 11:* 148, 1960.

Chapter 8

SPERMATOGENESIS

THE PROLIFERATION of large numbers of spermatogonia and the successive changes in morphology of these cells and chromosomal pattern, ultimately leading to the production of spermatozoa is the process spoken of as *spermatogenesis.* It is indeed one of the most unusual physiological processes in the human body.

"The prodigality of sperm production is a striking phenomenon," writes Hartman.[1] "Thus in the reproductive lifetime of an average man he will discharge four hundred billion sperms or a billion for every ovum that leaves a woman's ovary. No satisfactory explanation of the phenomenon has been offered."

Spermatogenesis is comparable to oogenesis in the female, each representing sexual maturity in the respective sexes. Spermatogenesis differs from oogenesis in that it may persist in old age and is a continuous process until death.[2] Nutrition, endocrines and some unknown conditions may interfere with the production of sperm but if inherently normal no interference occurs.[3]

In aged men degeneration of the seminiferous tubules may occur. In such cases it is believed that degenerative changes, especially of the blood vessels, interferes with sperm production. It is interesting to note that a striking feature of the testis of the aged is a thickening of the basement membrane and the presence of small round cells instead of spermatogenic cells. This histologic picture closely resembles the histology seen in undeveloped testes of young males. The histologic picture of the testes of the aged dying from accidental death is not essentially different from that of younger men. The aging process in the male gonad is not as marked or uniform as it is in the chronological years of aging in the female gonad. It is a variable factor and differs markedly in individuals. For further elaboration of this phase of spermatogenesis the reader is referred to Chapter 14 (The Testis in the Aged).

Spermatogenesis commences with the advent of puberty. At this time the lining cells of the seminiferous tubules undergoes a complex type of stratification and the seminiferous tubules increases in diameter with distinct formation of a lumen. Two types of cells can be identified: the Sertoli cells and the spermatogenic cells. The Sertoli cells, also spoken of as supporting or sustentacular cells, are not germinal cells even though they develop at the same time as the spermatogenic cells, from the indifferent epithelium of the seminiferous tubule. They serve as structural and supporting cells and are believed to nourish the spermatids. It is about at this time that the interstitial cells of Leydig now become differentiated. Shortly after puberty, characteristic Leydig cells develop in great numbers. In fact at this stage they are present in far greater numbers than are seen later in the adult testis. The origin of the germ cells present at puberty, are undoubtedly the result of hormonal stimulation (gonadotropin) but the exact mechanism is unknown. Sniffen[4,5] believes that from a purely morphologic standpoint, one would suspect that both the germ cells and the Sertoli cells stem from the undifferentiated nuclei of the tubular syncytium.

Spermatogenesis[6,7,8,9,10] is accomplished step by step in an orderly fashion. At first there are a great number of germ cells, the spermatogonia, situated in four to eight layers between the basement membranes and the lumen of the seminiferous tubule. The spermatogonia are round or cuboidal cells with a diameter of about 12 microns. They have round and highly chromatic nuclei. These cells undergo active proliferation, enlarge and form primary spermatocytes, which are found more centrally in the lumen. Upon attaining full development, the primary spermatocyte divides into two secondary spermatocytes and this phase is spoken of as the period of maturation, which is completed when early secondary spermatocyte divide to produce two spermatids. The spermatids are smaller than the primary and secondary spermatocytes and have a diameter of about 9 microns. They are within the lumen, undergo no further division, and are seen to be attached to the Sertoli cells, from which it is believed they derive their nourishment.

Of interest in this orderly process is *that in the two maturation divisions by which one primary spermatocyte gives rise to four spermatids,* a change in cell division occurs. This alteration from the usual mitotic division is spoken of as *Meiosis.* In this manner the number of chromosomes contained in a germ cell is reduced by half, so that spermatogonia and primary spermatocytes containing the full 48 chromosomes characteristic of all somatic cells of the human species produce mature germ cells containing half that number.* Thus the sex chromosomes* in the male as represented by X and Y chromosomes in half of the secondary spermatocytes, spermatids and spermatozoa contain the X chromosome and half the Y chromosome. It follows that if such halving of the chromosomal number did not occur in mature sex cells, subsequent fertilization of an ovum by a spermatozoa would produce a cell with double the normal number of chromosomes.

Further morphological differentiation occurs to the spermatid, which ultimately becomes a highly differentiated spermatozoan. In this alteration the nucleus becomes the sperm head while portions of the Golgi, mitochondrial and cytoplasmic material become the tail and the sheath. With full differentiation, spermatozoa become detached from the Sertoli cells and migrate rapidly to the epididymis. In histologic preparations of the testis few if any mature sperms are found lying free within the lumen of the seminiferous tubules. Varying degrees of activity are found along the tubules and a large section of the testis can be found to be in an intermediate state of spermatogenesis. This has been compared to the activity of renal glomeruli which shifts the working load to different tubules, leaving others in comparative states of rest.

Spermatogenesis is a continuous process in man and tremendous numbers of sperm cells are proliferated during the life of the normal male.[11] The mature spermatozoa are carried into the coiled epididymis where they are stored until such time as the orgasm (ejaculation) is accomplished. Observations tend to confirm the belief that the spermatozoa are immobile while retained

---

*The normal human chromosome number has now been established at 46. This number denotes 22 pairs of autosomes and 2 sex chromosomes, paired in the female (XX) and unpaired in the male (XY).[41, 42]

in the testis and are relatively quiescent while stored in the epididymis.[12] The spermatozoa are believed to be propelled to the epididymis by the cells lashing movement which motion begins when the sperm cell meets the secretion from the accessory glands. Once the spermatozoa reach the epididymis, they appear to undergo a progressive physiologic maturation during which their capacity for mobility and fertility increases. The epididymis is a single coiled tube approximately 18 feet long. It is not definitely known how long it takes for the passage of spermatozoon through the epididymis, but it is estimated to take about 10-12 days.* This movement is not entirely understood. Spermatozoa retained in the epididymis because of lack of ejaculation disintegrate and are reabsorbed. Some sperm are stored in the ductus deferens but contrary to a former belief are *not* stored in the seminal vesicles. The physiology and pharmacology of the epididymis is still an area not completely understood. We do not know, or at least have only fragmentary knowledge of what changes occur to the spermatozoa in their passage through the duct system.**

---

*Hartman[47] has recently estimated that spermatogenesis in man is completed in 48 days and that 12 days are required for the passage of sperms through the male genital tract. This determination was accomplished by marking spermatogonia with radioactive isotopes.

**The determination of fructose in semen has received considerable attention in the past decade. This unusual sugar is believed to be secreted by the seminal vesicles and is dependent on the presence of normal testosterone production, and contributes toward sperm motility. Deficient fructose production points indirectly to deficient testosterone production and Nowakowski[19] used evaluation of fructose of the semen as a measure of androgen activity and his curve, set up according to decades of life, is similar to the curve evaluated by Segal and Nelson,[20] namely a gradual decline with aging until 60 years, but with a relative constant value thereafter. The reader is referred to the excellent and exhaustive investigations of Mann *et al.*,[21] who clearly enunciate the significance of fructose as the natural energy subtrate for sperm in many mammals, including the mouse, rabbit, guinea pig, hamster, stallion, goat, bull, boar, ram and man. Fructose, according to these workers, is produced by the accessory sex organs under the influence of both androgen and gonadotropin. It is believed, based on strong experimental evidence, that seminal fructose is made available to the sperm at the moment of ejaculation, and prior to this time, the sperm, non-motile within the vas, must get along on their intracellular reserve.[22] This source of energy is mainly glucose, and the resulting glycolysis would give rise to copious quantities of lactic acid, reducing the pH and inhibiting sperm motility.

Indeed it has been postulated that it is quite possible that "some spermatozoa may not survive the environment of the epididymis and that abnormal conditions in that environment may, in some individuals at least, result in undue germ-cell destruction, to the point where the number of cells appearing in the ejaculate is not representative of the functional state of the germinal epithelium as determined by the biopsy."[12] These workers also raise the question as to whether the rate of progression of the sperm through the epididymis to the ductus deferens is steady and unrelated to the "demand" for spermatozoa or is the progression conditioned simply by the pressure from behind of spermatozoa produced at a steady rate from the germinal epithelium. Mac Leod[11] and Heim have demonstrated that in three ejaculates obtained at 24 hour intervals there is a progressive fall in the total number of cells. However, in an individual with high sperm count at the beginning, this does not necessarily mean a fall in potential fertility. Farris[18] confirmed this quantitative data.*

"According to modern views," states Cross,[17] "the motility of spermatozoa is of critical importance only for the penetration of the ovum at fertilization. The long journey from the seminiferous tubule to the ampulla of the Fallopian tube is probably effected at all stages by contractile mechanisms in the male and female genital tracts. Undoubtedly much of the contractile activity is independent of central nervous control, but there is reason to suppose that transportation of sperms is assisted by central nervous mechanisms set in motion by the sexual stimulation attending coitus. The hypothalmus may influence these processes in two ways: by autonomic pathways to the reproductive organs, especially via the sympathetico-adrenal system, and by its control of the secretion of oxytocin from the neurohypophysis."

Once the sperm cells reach the vasa deferentia, the further transportation is brought about by the powerful contractions of the muscular arrangement of these ducts. Contractions are rhythmically followed by expansions, which act as pumps and suck or draw out more sperm cells from the epididymis. Finally when

*The reader interested in more information on this phase of spermatogenesis is referred to the bibliography found at the end of this chapter.

they reach the urethra through the ejaculatory ducts, they are rapidly accelerated and emitted through the external urethral meatus. The male with rapid and successive ejaculations in repeated coitus at short intervals, diminishes the amount of seminal fluid. In fact, microscopically such a specimen would contain few normal and active sperms, and mostly abnormal and immature sperms. It is for this reason that evaluation of the semen should be made only after some restraint in coitus. However a man with a sperm count of 40-150 million per cc, after 2-4 days of continence, does not necessarily increase the fertility potential by increasing the period of continence and his sperm count.[15]

Following the ejaculation spermatozoa have a variable period of viability depending mainly upon temperature influences. At room temperature in a neutral container (not condom) they may remain viable for the first 3-5 hours. Some mobility may be noted at the end of 24 hours. Mobility may exist for 1-3 days in the uterus and fallopian tubes but ceases after a few hours in the vagina.

Man produces enormous numbers of spermatozoa during his life span. The average sperm count is 120,000,000 per cc, but fertility may occur with counts as low as 50,000,000 per cc. In Hotchkiss,[23] Breener and Greenley's series of 200 fertile men, 52 had counts of less than 60,000,000 per cc; in MacLeod's[11] series of 1,000 fertile men, 29% had less than 60 million per cc, 16% had less than 40 million, and 2% had less than 10 million sperm per cc. Of singular interest often over emphasized is the question of mobility and morphology of the spermatozoa. It is apparent from research studies that no clearly defined standards can be established which would separate the infertile male from the fertile male. What is most obvious is that men differ from one another in the sperm count but also that certain fluctuations occur in each male and this means that no diagnosis of infertility should be based upon one examination. These fluctuations, as Hotchkiss has pointed out, and quoted by Kirwin,[24] may be caused by one or all factors: (1) losses in the collection of the specimens; (2) errors inherent in laboratory techniques for analyzing the semen; (3) external and abnormal influences such as frequency of coitus, illness, etc.; and (4) physiological variations which are as yet not recognized. As emphasized by Hotchkiss,[6] each man holds to a certain pattern which is followed within certain limitations if the specimen is collected under standard conditions.

It may be useful to recall that the formation, output and composition of the semen, as found in the ejaculate, is not the result of one endocrine gland. It is the result of the composite action of several endocrine glands, most important of which are the testis and the pituitary gland. The anterior hypophysis exerts an influence on the testes, in an indirect manner, through interaction with other endocrine glands such as the adrenal cortex and the thyroid gland.

Routine investigation of fertility in the male does not necessarily require elaborate tests or complicated examinations. Semen analysis is a procedure which can be done in the physician's office, "the most important requirements are time and inclination."[6] For a detailed description of the method of collection of the semen specimen and semen analysis the reader is referred to any standard textbook on this subject. It suffices to say at this point that when one semen specimen proves defective, the physician should refrain from a final opinion until other specimens have been examined and that even if the seminal specimen appears satisfactory complete urologic investigation should be carried on.

The sperm count is a useful test for the evaluation of fertility in the male. The underlying cause of azoospermia or oligospermia cannot be determined by the sperm count alone. Additional information can and must be obtained by means of testis biopsy.

The male with consistently low sperm counts, with high percentage of abnormal spermatozoa and certainly one with no spermatozoa in the ejaculate should have the benefit of testicular biopsy. It should be emphasized, however, that *this is not a substitute* for a semen analysis. Indeed the testes biopsy and the semen analysis should be studied together, for one supplements the other. Testicular biopsy, first performed by Hotchkiss,[6] has in recent years received great impetus as an aid in determining the basic cause of an azoospermia or marked oligospermia. It is a simple procedure and permits excellent opportunity for a study

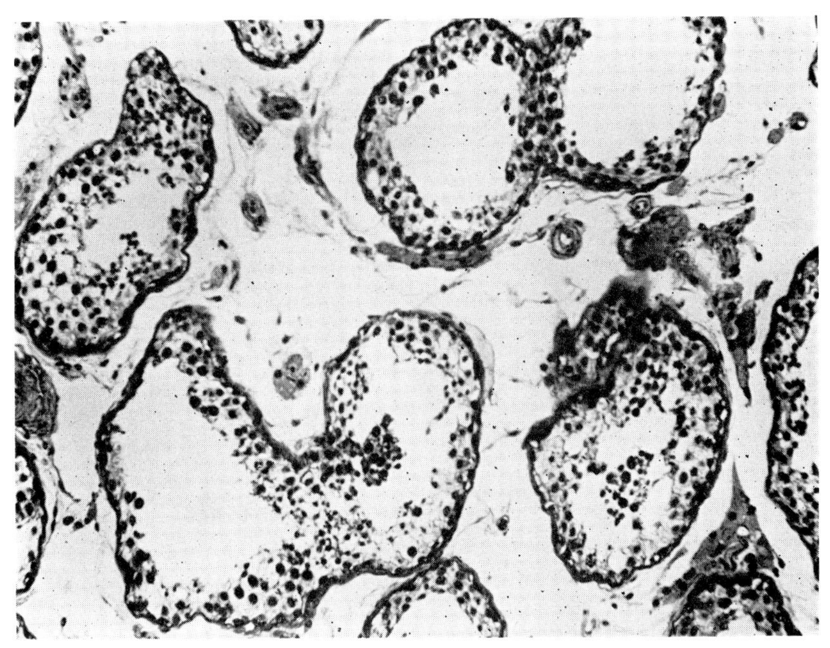

FIG. 14. Photomicrograph of testicular biopsy of 31 year old man, whose repeated seminal specimens showed azoospermia. This is a typical example of spermatogenic arrest, cause unknown, in which the process of sperm maturation is halted at one of the immature stages. In this case spermatogenesis is arrested at the spermatid stage.

of the microscopic pathology of the testicle in problems of infertility.

Some criticize the procedure in that they claim it does not give a picture of the testicle as a whole. Nevertheless it is of great value, particularly in (1) spermatogenic arrest; (2) peritubular fibrosis; and (3) germinal cell aplasia. Engle[25] states that, "The overall impression obtained from an examination of testis biopsies from cases with oligospermia is that there is a reduced rate of spermatogenesis. The tubules of the testes which produce a small number of sperm have all the components of the normal testis. Each cell is represented in proper proportion but all apparently in reduced numbers. Even though there are an abundance of tubules with all stages of spermatogenesis, the spermatids may not mature into spermatozoa. In the normal testis free spermatozoa are rarely seen in the lumens of the tubule. In testis biopsies of patients with oligospermia the spermatozoa frequently are found as free cells in the lumen of the tubule. The spermatozoa are apparently not undergoing the needed maturation within, or in contact with the cytoplasm of the sustentacular cell of Sertoli. In certain cases with a high percentage of abnormal spermatozoa, developmental abnormalities can be seen in the tubule. Distortions of cell division and abnormal nuclear structure are frequent. The spermatid nucleus may be very large, or the nucleus may be elongated with a beaded appearance." The testis biopsy is indeed a valuable aid in the detection of sterility, due to spermatogenic arrest.

Peritubular Fibrosis.—The most common cause of azoospermia is due to blockage of the duct system of the testis. The seminiferous tubules may undergo atrophy, with thickening and hyalinization of the tubule. This is not uncommon even in young males, although atrophy and fibrosis is most common in the old age group. The basic cause is not known and Engle is of the opinion that it is not of endocrine or nutritional origin. The process unfortunately is irreversible and there is no present evidence that its course can be arrested. It has frequently been noted among males with histories of severe infections, orchitis, testicular trauma, torsion or other lesion which would seriously interfere with the vascular supply of the testicle; yet in many cases no apparent basis or explanation of the underlying pathology can be found.

Germinal Aplasia. This condition is characterized by complete or almost complete absence of all cells of the germ cell line, including the parent cells, the spermatogonia. The seminiferous tubule has a normal contour and is not shrunken as in progressive tubular fibrosis. Sertoli cells are found in the tubules and the interstitial cells of Leydig are normal in shape and number. The etiology is unknown. Cases of germinal aplasia are found after x-radiation treatment of the testis, where the indicated dosage is sufficient to destroy the germ cells. Similar changes are seen in cryptorchid testicles of late adolescence.* Since the germinal

---

*A similar architectural pattern is seen in the testes of males suffering from Myotonia Dystrophica.[48,50]

epithelium does not exist, gonadotropic hormones are not utilized and the disorder is therefore characterized by elevated urinary levels of gonadotropins. This process like testicular fibrosis is irreversible and no therapy is indicated.

Spermatogenic Arrest.—This is the third type of testis pathology described by Engle,[25, 26, 27, 28] which also exhibits azoospermia of gonadal origin. It is a condition in which the process of spermatogenesis is arrested at the stage of primary spermatocyte, with the result that few or no sperm are produced. The large primary spermatocyte is easily identified. It is the largest cell present with a distinct cytoplasm and large, distinct nucleus. The arrested cells fragment and slough into the lumen of the tubules. The underlying cause is not known, but it has been suggested that it may be due to defects in the mechanisms of chromosomal synapse and division, or failure of the Sertoli cells to provide needed nutrition for spermatogenesis. Defective action of the gonadotropic hormone has also been suggested as an explanation of the disorder. In this condition the levels of urinary gonadotropins is usually normal.

It follows from the previous discussions that in men whose seminal specimens repeatedly show azoospermia, the evaluation of the testis is of paramount importance. In addition to the previously discussed disorders at the site of "manufacture" of sperm, some mechanical disturbance in the normal conveyance system of the sperm may be the underlying etiological agent. Thus it follows that in occlusion or absence of efferent ducts, the spermatogenic process is seriously hindered.

In Nelson's[29] series of cases, 22.8% revealed varying degrees of spermatogenic activity on testicular biopsy and in each instance demonstrated some defect, always bilateral, in the epididymis, vas deferens or both. Bilateral occlusion of the seminal ducts as a cause of azoospermia must not be minimized. The occlusion, usually due to gonorrheal vaso-epididymitis, may occur at any point in the efferent duct system but it is said to be found most frequent at the base of the epididymis and/or beginning of the vas deferens. It may be due to gonorrhea the result of post traumatic inflammation, congenital hyperplasia or vasectomy.

Of singular interest is that in the majority of such cases testicular biopsy reveals spermatogenesis rated as excellent or good and definitely falling into the category of normality. Occasionally but rarely, spermatogenesis will appear impaired and the histologic picture closely resembles that of "progressive peritubular sclerosis." It is believed that the fibrosis of the peritubular tissues, with thickness of the basement membrane and tunica propria interferes with normal nutrition of the germ cells.

In congenital bilateral absence of seminal ducts, a condition which may involve any part of the male efferent duct system from rete tubules through vasa efferentia, epididymis and vas deferens, the spermatozoa cannot be delivered even though they are being "manufactured." Testicular biopsy in the majority of such cases demonstrates excellent spermatogenesis. Such males could become fertile if the delivery of the spermatozoa could be affected. Michelson[30] and Hotchkiss[6] state that in such cases where the biopsy shows spermatogenesis to be essentially normal, the prognosis for fertility is fair, since anastomosis around the obstruction may reconstruct the channel for transportation of the sperm. If testicular biopsy reveals a serious defect of spermatogenesis (or severe peritubular fibrosis) permanent sterility is almost a certainty. The administration of testosterone propionate in high daily doses over a prolonged period of time (despite the immediate depression of spermatogenesis) followed by a "rebound" may offer some relief for these males.[31,32,33,34,35,36] This still awaits confirmation.*

At one time it was believed that occlusion of the vas deferens in old men and animals caused atrophy of the seminiferous tubules and hyperplasia of the interstitial cells of Leydig, the latter

*"The practice of giving large doses of testosterone to selected infertile males in order to elicit the rebound phenomenon has now extended over a period of nearly 10 years."[27] Charney[37] selects only those patients whose biopsies show a reversible lesion, defined as one in which the seminiferous tubules are of average size, contain normal though incompletely matured spermatogenic epithelium, and are enveloped by a membrana propia of thin collagenous fibers. In addition he rejects patients with a history of illness that might have disturbed spermatogenesis, if physical examination suggests the presence of first degree or second degree hypogonadism, if the testes are not normal in size and consistency and if the urine shows a reduced excretion of either gonadotropin or 17-ketosteroids.

resulting in increased secretion of androgenic hormone and rejuvenation. The reader will recall that Steinach[38] advocated the practice of vasectomy for rejuvenation of men and animals. This has been carefully disproven by Moore[39] who clearly demonstrates that not only is spermatogenesis not stopped by obstruction or absence of the seminal ducts, but also that the interstitial cells of Leydig do not undergo hyperplasia.

Congenital defects, such as absence can be determined clinically and the diagnosis suspected by careful palpation of the scrotum and its contents. This examination should first be performed with the patient lying down when a careful effort is made to palpate the upper portion of the scrotum. With the patient in the erect position the examiner must then thread the contents of the scrotum through the palpating fingers to determine the presence or absence of a palpable vas on either side.

I quite agree with Sohval,[40] who states, "A certain amount of confusion exists in the literature concerning the effects of experimental vasoligation and vasectomy. This is probably due to extraneous factors introduced by imperfect surgical technique. Accidental compromise of blood and nerve supply may induce severe degenerative changes in the testis which may be incorrectly attributed to obstruction of the vas deferens alone."

Experimental evidence tends to confirm the belief that vasectomy does not destroy completely the gametogenic function of the testis. Histologic examination of testes subjected to vasoligation reveal that many of the seminiferous tubules contain gametogenic cells. Some of the tubules do degenerate and it is assumed that the tubules alternately degenerate and repair.

As early as 1903 it was reported that vasoligation would destroy the spermatogenic tissue of the testis and lead to hypertrophy of the interstitial cells of Leydig. This gave rise to the hypothesis of rejuvenation in 1920 in which it was contended that (1) vasoligation of domestic animals and man destroys the germinal epithelium but increases the cells of Leydig, (2) the increase in number and size of the interstitial cells of Leydig produces an increased amount of male sex hormone, and (3) this release of increased androgens would "rejuvenate" the depleted male. The actual effect of vasectomy, other than sterilization, is still not fully understood.

Surgical correction of male sterility has made tremendous strides since Hagner[43] first outlined his operative procedure for anastomosis of the epididymis and vas deferens. Quinby[44] and Lespinasse[45] wrote extensively on the surgical correction of male sterility. O'Conor,[46] a former resident under Quinby, has reported on this phase of male sterility and the interested reader is urged to read the complete original article which is an instructive resume of the subject. O'Conor reviews 157 patients who presented themselves with complete azoospermia and in whom surgical exploration or corrective surgery was performed. In most instances the pathogenesis was the result of fibrous tissue, found in a single area or in multiple areas. This fibrosis was confined to the lumen of the vas in its scrotal and inguinal portion but most frequently in the lower portion of the globus minor and the most proximal portion of the vas.

"The diagnosis and indication for surgical intervention in these are not always entirely clear," states O'Conor.[46] "One should obtain a very careful history of the underlying problem and investigate the psychic element concerned with the sterile marriage before offering any optimistic outlook as to improvement by surgery." O'Conor speaks against frequent closed testicular biopsy and advocates scrotal exploration for careful inspection of the epididymis and vas.

Where surgery is indicated, the operative intervention is directed toward (a) uniting or anastomosing the vas and the epididymis, (b) anastomosis of the vas with individual epididymal tubules, (c) anastomosis of the vas deferens to a spermatococele, and (d) anastomosis of the cut ends of the vasa in an attempt to reestablish continuity of the lumen. O'Conor and his associates have in cases where complete occlusion of the distal portions of both vasa preclude any possibility of reanastomosis, devised a new procedure. In this technique the free and cut ends of both vasa are brought into the midline of the scrotum where they are allowed to empty into an inverted skin pouch. This reservoir can then be tapped for purposes of artificial insemination.

SUMMARY

(1) Spermatogenesis in the male is comparable to oogenesis in the female.

(2) Spermatogenesis is of a longer duration than oogenesis.

(3) The gametogenic mechanism of mature sperm consists of (a) preliminary stage of cell proliferation, (b) a period of cellular growth, (c) final stage of maturation in which the last two cellular divisions result in a sexual gamete with but one-half of the original number of chromosomes.

(4) Testicular histology can be altered by congenital anomalies, neoplasia inflammation, thermal and chemical influences and specific extra gonadal influences, all of which influence spermatogenesis.

(5) Testicular biopsy serves as an accurate index to the status of testicular histology.

(6) Sperm counts are important ancillary procedures for evaluation of testicular function.

(7) Hormonal influences are of specific importance in spermatogenesis. Thus the adenohypophysis responds to decreased or increased amounts of circulating gonadal hormone, establishing a reciprocal biologic balance of the pituitary-gonadal axis.

(8) Surgical correction of male sterility is indicated where there has been an interference with the continuity and/or patency of the lumen of the vas.

REFERENCES

1. Hartman, G. C.: *In Sex and Internal Secretions,* Allen, E., editor. 2nd Edition. Williams and Wilkins, Baltimore, M. D., 1958.
2. Engle, T. E.: The life history of the human testis. *J. Urol., 74:* 379, 1955.
3. Engle, T. E., and Jailer, J. W.: Endocrinology in Urology. In Campbell, M.: *Urology.* Vol. 3, pp. 1667-1700, W. B. Saunders Co., Philadelphia and London, 1954.
4. Sniffen, R. C.: The testis. 1. The normal testis. *Arch. Path., 50:* 259, 1950.
5. Sniffen, R. C.: Histology of the normal and abnormal testis at puberty. *Ann. New York Acad. Sci., 55:* 1952.
6. Hotchkiss, R. S.: Fertility in Men: *A Clinical Study of the Causes, Diagnosis and Treatment of Impaired Fertility in Men.* Lippincott, Philadelphia, 1944.

7. Howard, R. P., Sniffen, R. C., Simmons, F. A., and Albright, F.: Testicular deficiency; a clinical and pathologic study. *J. Clin. Endocrinol., 10(2):* 121-186, 1950.
8. Howard, R. P. Simmons, F. A., and Sniffen, R. C.: Differential diagnosis in male sterility. *J. Fertility and Sterility, 2(2):* 95-114, 1951.
9. MacLeod, J.: Semen quality in one thousand men of known fertility and in eight hundred cases of infertile marriage. *J. Fertility and Sterility, 2(2):* 115-139, 1951.
10. Simmons, F. A.: *Clinical Interpretation of the Semen Analysis Conference of Diagnosis in Sterility.* E. T. Engle, Ed. Thomas, Springfield, 1945.
11. MacLeod, J., and Heim, L. M.: Characteristics and variations in the semen specimens in 100 normal men. *J. Urol., 54:* 474, 1945.
12. Mason, K. E., and Shaver, S. L.: Some functions of the caput epididymis. *Ann. of the N. Y. Acad. of Sciences,* Vol. 55, p. 585, 1952.
13. Toothill, M. C., and Young, W. C.: The time consumed by spermatozoa in passing through the ductus epididymis of the guinea pig as determined by means of India ink injections. *Anat. Rec., 50:* 95-107, 1931.
14. Montagna, W., and Hamilton, J. B.: Histological studies of human testes. I. The distribution of lipids. *Anat. Rec., 109:* 635,-660, 1951.
15. MacLeod, J., and Gold, R. Z.: The kinetics of human spermatogenesis as revealed by changes in the ejaculate. *Ann. of the N. Y. Acad. of Sciences,* Vol. 55, p. 707, 1952.
16. MacLeod, J., and Heim, L. M.: Characteristics and variations in the semen specimens in 100 normal men. *J. Urol., 54:* 474, 1945.
17. Cross, E.: Quoted by Lowsley, O. S., and Kirwin, T. J.: *Clinical Urology.* 3rd Edition. Vol. 1. Williams & Wilkins Co., Baltimore, 1956.
18. Farris, E. J.: *Human Fertility.* The Author's Press, White Plains, N. Y., 1950.
19. Nowakowski, H.: *Acta. Endocrinol. Supplement., 31:* 117-148, 1957.
20. Segal, S . J., and Nelson, W. O.: *Initiation and Maintenance of Testicular Function.* Conference on Recent Progress in the Endocrinology of Reproduction. Edited by Loyd, C. W. Academy Press Inc., New York and London, 1959.
21. Mann, T., and Lutwak-Mann, C.: Secretory function of male accessory organs in mammals. *Physiol. Rev., 31:* 27, 1951.
22. Bishop, W. D.: In discussion of presentation: Gassner, F. X., Hill, H. J., and Sulzberger, B. A.: Relationship of seminal fructose to testis function in the domestic animal. *J. Fertility and Sterility, 3:* 121, 1952.
23. Hotchkiss, R. S., Brunner, E. K., and Greenley, P.: Semen analysis of two hundred fertile men. *Am. J. Med. Sci., 196:* 362-84, 1938.
24. Lowsley, O. S., and Kirwin, T. J.: *Clinical Urology.* 3rd Edition, Vol. 1, Williams and Wilkins Co., Baltimore, 1956.

25. Engle, E. T.: The testis biopsy in infertility. *J. Urol., 57:* 789-798, 1947.
26. Engle, E. T.: Atypical cytology in testis biopsies. *J. Urol., 62:* 694, 1949.
27. Engle, E. T.: *Problems of Ageing.* 2nd Ed. Chap. 17. Cowdry, E. V., Ed. Williams and Wilkins Co., Baltimore, 1942.
28. Engle, E. T.: The cytological problem in spermatogenic arrest. Annals of *The New York Acad. Medicine,* Vol. 55, p. 73, 1952.
29. Nelson, W. O.: *Spermatogenesis in Testes of Men with Blocked or Absent Efferent Ducts. In Studies on Testis and Ovary, Eggs and Sperm.* Engle, E. T., Ed. Thomas, Springfield, 1952.
30. Michelson, L.: Treatment of azoospermia by vaso-epididymal anastamosis. *Tr. Soc. Study Sterility,* 1946.
31. Moore, C. R., and Price, D.: Some effects of testosterone and testosterone propionate in the rat. *Anat. Record., 71:* 59, 1938.
32. Heller, C. G., Nelson, W. O., Hill, I. B., Henderson, E., Maddock, W. O., Jungck, E. C., Pauleson, C. A., and Mortimore, G. E.: Improvement in spermatogenesis following depression of the human testis with testosterone. *J. Fertility and Sterility, 1:* 415, 1950.
33. Hurxthal, L. N., Burns, H. J., and Musulinn: Development of spermatogenesis in hypogonadism. *J. Clin. Endocrinol., 9:* 1245, 1949.
34. Heckel, N. J., Rosso, W. A., and Kestel, L.: Spermatogenic rebound phenomenon after administration of testosterone propionate. *J. Clin. Endocrinol., 11:* 235, 1951.
35. Heckel, N. J., and McDonald, J. H.: Further observations on the rebound phenomenon of the spermatogenic activity of the human testis following administration of testosterone propionate. *J. Fertility and Sterility, 3:* 49, 1952.
36. Charny, C. W.: Treatment of male infertility with large doses of testosterone. *J.A.M.A., 160:* 98, 1956.
37. Charny, C. W.: The use of androgens for human spermatogenesis. *J. Fertil. and Sterility, 10:* 557, 1959.
38. Steinach, E.: Biological methods against the process of old age. *Med. Jour. & Rec.,* Jan. 19, and Feb. 2, 1927.
39. Moore, C. R.: Biology of the Testis. *In Sex and Internal Secretion.* The Williams and Wilkins Co., Baltimore, 1939.
40. Sohval, A. R.: In Soffer's *Diseases on the Endocrine Glands.* Section on Gonads. Lea and Febiger, Philadelphia, 2nd Edition, 1956.
41. Ford, C. E., and Hamerton, J. L.: Chromosomes of man. *Nature, London, 178:* 1020-1023, 1956.
42. Tjio, J. H., and Levan, A.: Chromosome number of man. *Hereditas, 42:* 1-6, 1956.
43. Hagner, F. R.: Sterility in the male. *Surg. Gyn. & Obst., 52:* 330, 1931.
44. Quinby, W. C.: Sterility in the male: its operative treatment when due to bilateral epididymitis. *Boston M. & S. J., 155:* 539, 1906.

45. Lespinasse, N. D.: Obstructive sterility in the male. *J.A.M.A., 70:* 448, 1918.
46. O'Conor, V.: Surgical correction of male sterility. *Surg. Gyn. & Obst., 110:* 649, 1960.
47. Hartman, G. G.: A half century of research in reproductive physiology. *J. Fertility and Sterility, 12:* 1, 1961.
48. Clark, B. G., Shapiro, S., Monroe, R. G.: Myotonia atrophica with testicular atrophy; urinary excretion of interstitial cell-stimulating (lutenizing) hormone, androgens and 17-ketosteroids. *J. Clin. Endocr., 16:* 1235, 1956.
49. Sohval, A. R., Soffer, L. J.: Congenital familial testicular deficiency. *Am. J. Med., 14:* 328, 1953.
50. Ledwith, J. W., and Whipple, R. J.: Myotonia Dystrophica: A case report with sex chromatin studies. *Annals Int. Med., 54:* 113, 1961.

Chapter 9

CRYPTORCHISM

MUCH HAS BEEN written regarding cryptorchism. The literature is replete with varied and divergent opinions. "Cryptorchism has a two-fold etiology. It is caused either by an abnormality of the pathway through which the testis moves from the retroperitoneal space to the scrotum or by a defective propelling mechanism which fails to move the testis through a normal pathway to its destination."[1] What makes the problem of cryptorchism even more difficult is that this defect in travel may result from either a lack of stimulation to the testis or from an inherent defect of the testis whereby it is unable to respond to proper gonadotropic stimulation. In the former instance the basic cause is the pituitary, namely pituitary hypofunction (hypogonadotropism), and in the latter case the testis is structurally defective (hypogonadism), and is unable to respond to the proper gonadotropic stimulation.[2]

All are agreed that the testis must migrate to the scrotum, for if it does not travel to the scrotum the seminiferous tubules fail to mature and will not function properly. "Teleologically," states Sohval,[3] "the testis descends into the scrotum because this external location provides a lower temperature which is essential for future spermatogenesis." Thus when not in the scrotum, but in the inguinal canal or in the abdominal cavity, the testis is exposed to harmful influence of a higher temperature which deteriorates the germinal epithelium of the seminiferous tubules. This degeneration ultimately provides a small and atrophic testicle, despite the fact that there is no atrophy or deterioration of the interstitial cells of Leydig. This is confirmed by the fact that cryptorchism does not interfere with the preservation of the secondary sexual characteristics. In man the temperature of the scrotum is about

40° C lower than that of the abdomen. The seminiferous tubules do not develop or function properly unless the testis is situated in the lower most portion of the scrotum, under control of the thermo-regulator mechanism.

Mechanism of Descent.—The male gonad is derived from the mid-portion of the genital ridge on a level with the first and second lumbar vertebrae. During embryonic development, the gonad, except for a slender stalk called the *mesorchium,* lies free in the peritoneal cavity. The mesorchium anchors the testis to the anterior abdominal wall, and this fulcrum serves as a guide to the ultimate migration of the testis from the posterior abdominal wall to its scrotal destination.[4,5]

Early in embryonic life the gonad consists of two layers of germinal epithelium, a central, loose cell mass, and a peripheral compact mass. The central mass became more defined as an inner and outer portion and from the inner portion are later developed the seminiferous tubules. The tunica albuginea develops from the outer portion of the central mass and the visceral coat of the tunica vaginalis develops from the peripheral layer of cells.[6]

Actually the testis in early fetal life is a retroperitoneal structure, connected to the anterior abdominal wall by a fold of peritoneum, called the inguinal fold.[7,8] The inguinal fold fuses with a peritoneal fold of the anterolateral abdominal wall called the inguinal crest. Between these folds the gubernaculum testis appears as a band of musculofibrous tissue. This first occurs at about the third month of embryonic development. In time the lower portion of the gubernaculum becomes thicker while the upper portion becomes thinner and ultimately disappears.

The testis assumes a lower and lower position as the embryo develops so that by the third to fourth month as the embryo begins to straighten itself, the testis is at or near the internal inguinal ring. Further descent is accomplished by proliferation of the process vaginalis through the anterior abdominal wall and thereby forming the inguinal canal. It emerges at the external inguinal ring, ultimately reaching the bottom of the scrotum. At the eighth to ninth month, and sometimes not until birth, the testis descends behind the patent processus vaginalis to lie in its normal position at the bottom of the scrotum, which is now fully developed. The pouch of the peritoneum, which later becomes the tunica vaginalis, precedes the testis into the scrotum and later with full descent seals off the testicle and its appendages. At surgery, the undescended testis will usually be found just inside the inguinal ring, in the inguinal canal, or deflected from the external ring in various abdominal positions. Charney[1] and Wolgin emphasize that the descent of the testis is independent of the descent of the processus vaginalis and the testis neither pushes the processus vaginalis down in its descent, nor is it pulled down by it.

At birth, the normal testis is an oval structure averaging about 1.2 cm. in its greatest diameter. Histologically the tubules are small and completely filled with undifferentiated cells. For the first 5 days, it is possible to detect a few interstitial cells of Leydig which are believed to persist because of maternal chorionic gonadotropin stimulation. The testicle now begins to grow in direct proportion to the growth of the rest of the body so that at age 4 we see a different histological picture. At this age the tubules are about 65 microns in diameter and they now have a definite lumen with cells identified as spermatogonia lining the basement membrane. Three years later (age 7) the tubules measure 70 microns in diameter but there is little change in the cellular picture. At age 10 proof of sexual maturation is first detected as evidenced by (1) acceleration of tubular growth; (2) presence of mitotic figures; (3) presence of primary and secondary spermatocytes; and (4) interstitial cells of Leydig are again seen (now as a result of pituitary secretion). From this phase, development is rapid and by 12-14 years of age the seminiferous tubule assumes the adult appearance.

What about the testicle that does not descend? Data obtained by biopsy studies reveals that the spermatogenic elements of the undescended testis exhibit minimal degeneration changes before age 10. There are however definite changes after this age if the testicle is permitted to remain in its abnormal environment. Maturation fails to take place and degenerative changes now take place. The longer the testis remains outside the scrotum the greater are these changes and according to most authorities on this subject, the damage to the seminiferous tubules is proportionate to the duration of the undescended testicle and not to the degree of non-descent.[9,10,11] It follows that where the faulty descent is due to a defect in structure, such as in hypogonadism, such a testis will reveal evidence of a congenital subnormal gonad, characterized by a lack of tubular and cellular maturation. If due to a secondary hormonal defect, as in hypopituitarism, failure of descent is due to lack of gonadal or gonadotrophic stimulation. Such a testicle reveals a normal histologic appearance and if left alone may spontaneously descend or may descend after stimulation with chorionic gonadotropin administration.

Thus failure of descent may be attributed to (1) mechanical factors; (2) lack of hormonal stimulation; or (3) testicular

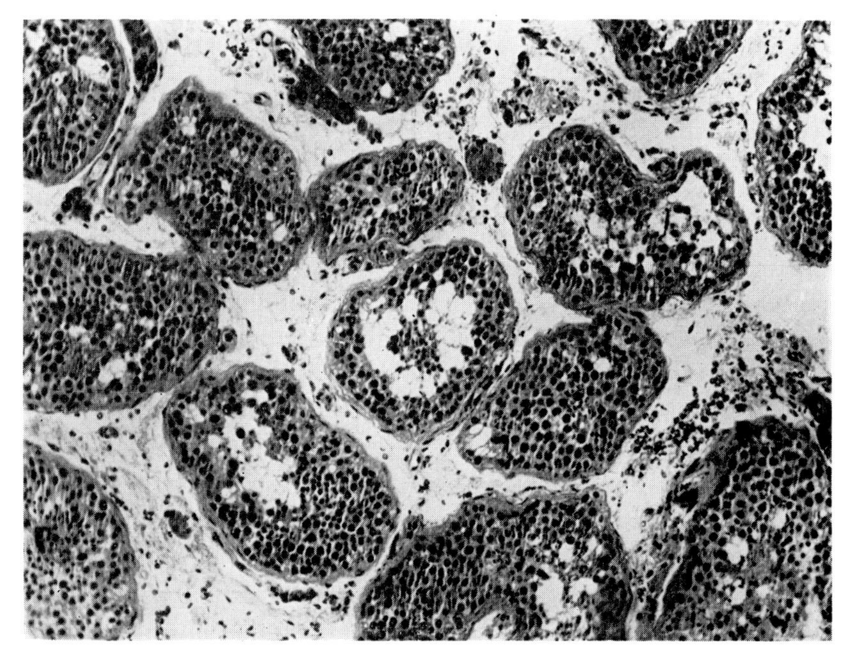

FIG. 15. Photomicrograph of section of undescended testicle of an adult (gross specimen measured 2.3 x 1.8 x 1 cm. and weighed 5 grams). Section demonstrates marked atrophy characterized by advanced fibrosis of basement membrane of the seminiferous tubules. Germinal maturation is arrested at 1° spermatocyte stage. Sertoli cells are well demonstrated.

deficiency prohibiting testicular response to hormonal stimulation.[10, 11, 12]

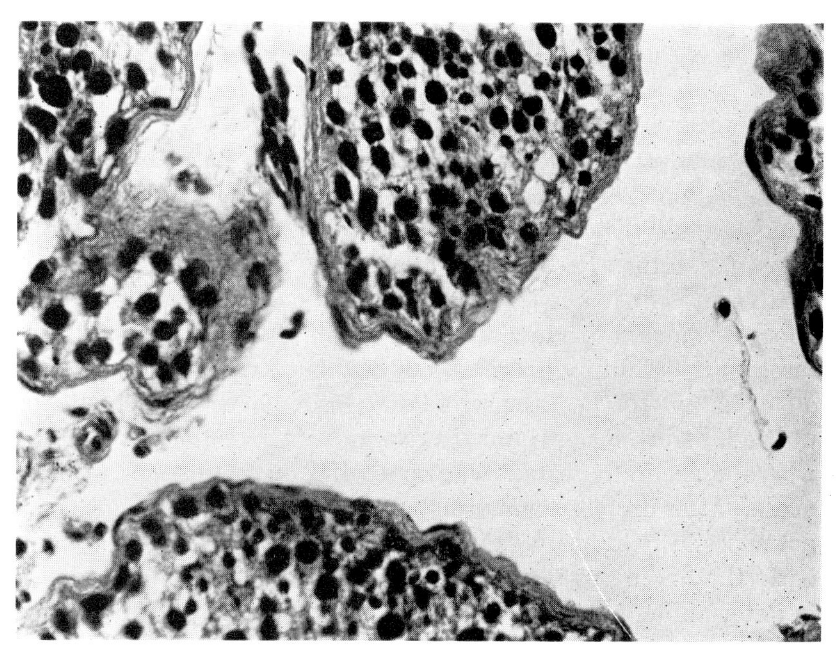

FIG. 16. Same as Figure 15—high power. This architectural pattern is similar to that seen in the testes of the aged. Note thickening of tunica propria.

Charney,[13] in a recent discussion of the spermatogenic potential of the undescended testis before and after treatment is quite pessimistic about the prevailing methods of treatment of cryptorchism and believes that the operative techniques, as practiced by most surgeons, yield better cosmetic than functional results. To quote Charney, "In the hands of most surgeons, orchiopexy fails to induce or to restore normal tubular function. Biopsies of a large number of testes which were brought into the scrotum by a variety of techniques fails to reveal a single instance of normal spermatogenesis. Admittedly, many of the operative techniques employed in inducing descent of the testis under observation are now considered out moded. Fixation of the testis to the inner surface of the thigh, as suggested by Thorek, is sufficiently damaging to interfere with its proper development, and the Bevan technique which depends primarily on retroperitoneal dissection yields results which are not much better." "However," continues Charney, "some of the biopsies reported were done on testes which were brought into the scrotum by techniques which are now considered acceptable."

It is interesting to note that many of these cases biopsied by Charney, had been recalled for follow up by their surgeons, and had been told that the results were excellent, even though on gross examination the appearance of the testis was indicative of failure. In this respect it is well to remember that in all post-operative check-ups a slight reduction in size or a fixed high position in the scrotum is uniformly diagnostic of disturbed spermatogenesis. In all cases as will be discussed later, testicular biopsy should be utilized, before surgery and after surgery. This is the only method whereby accurate evaluation of potential spermatogenesis can be made. After orchiopexy, normal size and position of the testis are not necessarily indicative of the function of the "fixed" testis. Similarly the finding of spermatozoa in the ejaculate is only of value in determining the spermatogenic value in the "fixed" testes (bilateral cryptorchism).

In addition to spermatogenesis of the undescended testicle, the problem of malignancy of the undescended testicle has been a moot subject for many years. In the light of our present knowledge one can only say that even if the testicle is placed in its normal postion it is still prone to possible malignant changes. This has aroused the question as to whether orchiopexy is an approved procedure, solely as a preventive measure against testicular carcinoma. Although the weight of evidence is in favor of an increased potential toward malignant degeneration of an undescended testicle, it is actually impossible to accurately estimate from available data the true incidence of such a complication in cryptorchidism. However if we are to accept the theory of testicular dysgenesis in the undescended testicle, as confirmed by testicular biopsy studies, it would be more logical to assume that such changes are responsible for neoplasia and not the ectopic position of the testis. This seems to be more accurate for the incidence of malignancy remains unchanged after orchiopexy, if orchiopexy is performed after tubular changes have occurred in the misplaced gonad. Sohval[9, 12, 14, 15] and others are of this opinion and believe testicular dysgenesis is the significant factor in testicular carcinoma.

"It would appear," states Lich,[18] "that the only consistent advantage of orchiopexy is to fill the totally or half empty scrotum and thus remove the obvious evidence in the eyes of the parent who feels that they have given the child an inadequate inheritance. The psychologic trauma of cryptorchidism is spoken of as an unequivocal fact. In the instance of bilateral cryptorchidism this could be true, but in unilateral retained testis this may be rightfully questioned. In questioning adults with unilateral nondescent there is most times little concern expressed over this abnormality and was equally of little disturbance during their youth. In children it often is apparent that any anxiety that exists on the part of the child is a direct reflection of the constant attention, concern and apprehension demonstrated by the parents. The inconspicuousness of cryptorchism in the child or adult is quite apparent by the rarity of its inclusion as a secondary diagnosis in general hospital charts."

This same author stresses the need of consideration of certain indications for secondary orchiopexy even though primary orchiopexy may be considered a debatable subject. "A symptomatic cryptorchid inguinal hernia should be repaired and a concomitant orchiopexy executed. If at hernioplasty there is a testis that cannot be placed easily in the scrotum the problem becomes one of leaving the testis in the inguinal position or in the scrotal neck or orchiectomy. If the opposite testis is normal and the testis in question is grossly abnormal or can be so demonstrated by immediate histologic study, orchiectomy is preferable. If the opposite testis is morphologically or functionally abnormal the testis in question should be left in the inguinal region for observation. In abnormally retained testes they should be removed if scrotal relocation is impossible, provided the opposite testis is normal; otherwise inguinal placement for observation."

Treatment.—The treatment of cryptorchism is either (a) hormonal or (b) surgical. Failure to descend after hormonal treatment usually indicates mechanical obstruction which requires surgery.[12, 15]

(a) Hormonal Treatment.—It is now more than a quarter of a century since hormonal treatment for cryptorchism was first inaugurated. As clearly defined by Charney[1] and Wolgin a discussion of the criteria for treatment should include indications as "the age at which treatment should be started and the clinical significance of spontaneous adequate fertility, elimination of possible potential focus of malignancy, correction of hernia if associated with cryptorchism and finally for avoidance of possible psychic disturbances which may be precipitated because of the genital anomaly." The latter at times may even lead to quasi-organic impotence.[26]

Unfortunately there is no universal agreement as to the age of initiating hormonal treatment or even when to operate. The reader must avoid following procedures which are now antiquated. For example, it was customary during the early part of the century for the surgeon to defer surgery until puberty. This was accepted as a general rule since it was then believed that by this age the testes would be sufficiently mature to respond to corrective surgery. It soon became apparent to the surgeon that there was as much need for functional correction as well as cosmetic, and that delay in permitting the testes to remain outside the scrotum until puberty, resulted in non-functioning testes.

With the introduction of chorionic gonadotropin hormone further changes in therapy of this genital anomaly took place. This anterior pituitary-like principal known as APL and pharmacologically as follutin-S is now universally used in cryptorchism, preferably at about 7-8 years of age and definitely before age 10. It is at the latter age that some workers have found that the non-scrotal testis lags in development and that it is disadvantageous to keep such a testicle in its abnormal position after age ten.

Deming[19] believes that theoretically at least the most favorable cases for the use of the hormone are the bilateral cryptorchids, because, "without obstruction to their course of descent, their most probable failure to descend was due to the deficiency of the hormone in utero. These are most difficult ones to treat primarily with surgery because of the short spermatic arteries. The testis has never migrated, and its artery, no matter what its origin has rarely had an opportunity to elongate sufficiently to reach the scrotum. The testis in these bilateral cases are less likely to show anatomical dysgenesis than the unilateral cryptorchid, and offer greater percentage of potential physiological normal development than unilateral cryptorchids. In the cases of unilateral cryptorchid, we have a different problem. Both testes have been theoretically subjected to equal opportunities for descent by the action of the hormones in utero, and it would not be expected that more gonadotropic hormone would induce a descent of these testes."

The dosage of gonadotropic hormone varies universally and this too has been a moot subject. The dosage has varied from small amount of 100 I.U. twice or three times weekly to 500 I.U. three times weekly. Robinson[20] and Engle tried 4000 to 5000 units of chorionic gonadotropin per day for three consecutive days and if descent did not occur by then they recommended surgery. Large doses of the hormone are to be avoided because if continued for over a long period of time, precocious sexual development occurs as well as premature union of epiphyses and psychic disturbance. Charney and Wolgin[1] recommend intramuscular administration of chorionic gonadotropin in doses averaging 500 I.U. three times weekly and if descent does not occur after 10,000 I.U. have been injected, hormonal treatment should be discontinued. These authors recommend the administration of thyroid substance only in the hypothyroid male, and although they discuss small doses of testosterone as a final endocrine test in doses of 15 to 30 mg. weekly for a total dosage of 300 mg., they are not enthusiastic about this form of therapy.

All who have had any experience in the hormonal treatment of cryptorchids are emphatic in the denial of its value in cases with ectopic testis, migratory testis, pseudo-cryptorchids, agenesis of testis, cryptorchids with large hernias and hydrocele and in all post puberty cases.

(b) Surgical Treatment.–Orchiopexy or surgical placement of the undescended testis into the scrotum was first attempted in

1820 by Rosenmerkel.[21] Because of most unsatisfactory results it remained in disrepute until 1899, when Bevan[22] first published the results of his improved technique. It was in the later article which also appeared in the *Journal of the American Medical Association* that he advocated bisection of all the structures of the cord except the vas deferns, deferential artery, and vein, in those cases in which the internal spermatic vessels are too short for scrotal placement. In 1918, he wrote in the *Surgical Clinics,* advocating the purse-string suture around the neck of the scrotum. Further stimulus was given to orchiopexy by Torek[23] who added the principal of fixation to Bevan's doctrine of mobilization. This two-stage orchiopexy was introduced independently by Keetley in England.[24, 25]

SUMMARY

It is well to emphasize that a child with one undescended testicle has every good reason of being a perfectly normal male as to sexuality and ability to procreate. However a child with bilateral undescended testicles will have normal sexual development, libido and potency but has only about a 10% chance of being able to reproduce. Prolonged retention of the testes out of the scrotum is damaging and always associated with a high incidence of congenital defectiveness. This defectiveness is often seen in the undescended mate as well. For this reason it is not advisable to assume that in an otherwise normal preadolescent boy, cryptorchism spontaneously cures itself in most instances.

Most authorities now agree that

(1) The undescended testicle probable is more apt to develop malignant degeneration than its scrotal mate;

(2) orchiopexy does not prevent malignant degeneration;

(3) the retained testis and scrotal testis develop equally during the first five years of life and thereafter the retained testis falls rapidly behind normal spermatogenesis;

(4) avoid whenever possible simultaneous bilateral orchiopexy because 10% of all post operative orchiopexies develop post operative testicular atrophy;

(5) a palpable inguinal testis should have the benefit of a hormonal trial;

(6) chorionic gonadotropin should be administered, preferably at 8-9 years of age, in relatively large doses (500 to 1,000 I.U.) either daily or three times weekly for a total of 10,000 I.U. If signs of precocious sexual development, such as growth of pubic hair and development of the penis, appear without progress in the descent of the testicle, treatment should be discontinued;

(7) testosterone propionate may be used in 10 mg. dosage, either alone or along with the chorionic gonadotropin. Signs of sexual precocity must be carefully watched for, since the giving of testosterone in excess is known to produce tubular damage, and finally;

(8) if success does not follow such a regime the only other therapy available is either (a) orchiopexy or (b) orchiectomy.

Leadbetter[27] has well summarized the surgery of the undescended testis in the following manner: "Undescended testes are treated surgically for four reasons: first, to correct an anatomical abnormality which may be embarassing to a growing child; second, to encourage the normal development of testes to produce sperm; third, to bring testicles into the scrotum so that possible tumor formation will be noted early; and, fourth, to correct associated congenital hernia."

REFERENCES

1. Charney, C. W., and Wolgin, W.: *Cryptorchism.* Hoeber-Harper, 1957.
2. Herbut, P. A.: *Urological Pathology.* Lea and Febiger, Philadelphia, 1952.
3. Sohval, A. R.: In Soffer's: *Diseases on the Endocrine Glands.* Lea and Febiger, Philadelphia, 2nd Edition, p. 464, 1956.
4. Arey, H. B.: *Developmental Anatomy.* W. B. Saunders, Philadelphia, 1948.
5. Gruenwald, P.: Development of Sex Cords in gonads of man and mammals. *Am. J. Anat., 70:* 359, 1942.
6. Jost, A.: Recherches sur la differenciation sexuelle de l'embryon de lapin. III Role des gonades foetales dans la differenciation sexuelle somatique. *Arch. Anat. Micr. et Morphol. Expér., 36:* 271, 1947.
7. Jones, H. J., Jr., and Scott, W. W.: *Hermaphroditism, Genital Anomalies and Related Endocrine Disorders.* Chapter 2, The Williams and Wilkins Co., Baltimore, 1958.
8. Arey, L. B.: *Developmental Anatomy.* W. B. Saunders, Philadelphia, 1948.

9. Sohval, A. R.: Testicular Dysgenesis as an etiological factor in cryptorchidism. *J. Urol., 72:* 693, 1954.
10. Wells, L. J.: Descent of the testis. *Surg., 14:* 436, 1943.
11. Moore, C. R., and Quick, W. J.: Scrotum as temperature regulator for testis. *Am. J. Physiol., 68:* 70, 1942.
12. McGregor, A. L.: The third inguinal ring. *Surg. Gynecol. and Obst., 49:* 273-309, 1929.
13. Charney, C. W.: The spermatogenic potential of the undescended testes before and after treatment. *J. Urol., 83:* 697, 1960.
14. Cooper, E.: The histology of the retained testis in the human subject at different ages, and its comparison wtih the scrotal testis. *J. Anat., 64:* 5, 1929.
15. Sohval, A. R.: The histopathology of cryptorchism. *Am. J. Med., 16:* 346, 1954.
16. Nelson, W. O.: Mammalian spermatogenesis: effect of experimental cryptorchidism in the rat and non-descent of the testis in man. Recent Progress in Hormone Research, 6129, 1951.
17. Sniffen, R. C.: Histology of the normal and abnormal testis at puberty. *Ann. of the New York Acad. of Sciences,* Vol. 55, p. 609, 1952.
18. Lich, R.: Cryptorchidism. *The American Surg., 22:* 2, 1956.
19. Deming, C. L.: Hormonal and surgical bases for treatment of undescended testis. *Am. J. Surg., 38:* 186-191, 1937.
    Indications for hormonal treatment of cryptorchidism. *J. Urol.,* Vol. 77, No. 3, March, 1957.
20. Robinson, J. N., and Engle, E. T.: Some observations on cryptorchid testis. *J. Urol., 71:* 726, June, 1954.
21. Rosenmerkel, J. F.: *Ueber die Radicalcur des in der Weiche Liegenden Testikels bei Nicht Descensus Desselben.* J. Lindauer, Munich, 1820.
22. Bevan, A. D.: Surgical treatment of undescended testicle. Further Contribution. *J.A.M.A., 41:* 178-724, 1903.
23. Torek, F.: Orchiopexy for undescended testicle. *Ann. Surg., 94:* 97, 1931.
24. Keetley, C. B.: Temporary fixation of the testis to thigh. A series of 25 cases operated on for undescended testis. *Lancet, 2:* 279-281, 1905.
25. Wershub, L. P.: Orchiopexy: A Critique. *J. Urol., 60:* 631, 1948.
26. Wershub, L. P.: *Sexual Impotence in the Male.* Thomas, Springfield, 1959.
27. Leadbetter, W. F.: In correspondence section. *J.A.M.A., 174:* 1653, 1960.

Chapter 10

HYPOGONADISM

FOR CENTURIES it has been known that besides its reproductive capacity the testes exerts an entirely independent influence upon the human organism. The ancients[1] were aware of the marked changes that occurred when men or male animals were castrated. Such humans fail to develop secondary male characteristics, have no sexual power, and physically closely resemble the female. Functional deficiencies may also occur in moderate or severe forms of hypogonadism other than as a result of castration.

In this chapter we will confine our thoughts to *hypogonadism,* or decrease in the function of the male gonads, bearing in mind that the gonads are primarily concerned with (1) producing androgens and (2) producing sperm. The status of the gonads therefore is of singular importance to the clinician for these two functions of male gonads are essential for the propagation of mankind.

When the gonad does not function properly, i.e., has a *deficiency of testicular function,* sexual behavior is disturbed or eliminated, and if function is faulty before puberty, there will be an interference in the growth of the secondary sex organs. In addition gonadal status influences skeletal growth and muscular development. When one considers the complexity of spermatogenesis, response and sensitivity of the germinal epithelium to various physical, thermal and chemical agents, as well as the vulnerability of the testes to trauma, it is surprising that more males are not victims of some pathological physiology of the testis.

One would assume that the best means of determining whether the gonads are functioning properly would be by examination of the genitalia. The status of the external genitalia is dependent to a great extent upon the secretion of androgens which is manifested by normal masculine development. However the size of the testicles is a variable factor, as is the size of the penis. In cases of hypogonadism where the testicles are obviously small and atrophic some index of gonadal status can be determined by clinical examination. At least suspicion of inadequate gonadal status should be aroused by the smallness of the testes. But testicular size in itself does not necessarily indicate the amount of androgen production or gonadal status.*

Heller[2] and Nelson in a careful classification of male hypogonadism emphasize that on clinical grounds alone it is often impossible to determine whether hypogonadism is the result of testicular failure or of primary pituitary failure leading to testicular failure. This distinction is important for the type and length of treatment is dependent upon such differentiation. They recommend the therapeutic test with chorionic gonadotropin. This consists of the administration of 750 international units of chorionic gonadotropin intramuscularly twice weekly for three weeks. If a response (urinary gonadotropins) is elicited, the authors refer to the status as hypogonadotropic hypogonadism. If no response is elicited the patient is then definitely hypogonadal. Primary hypogonadism is not influenced by injection of gonadotropins (APL) since in these cases the pituitary is intact and there is already an *overabundance* or *adequate supply* of gonadotropins appearing in the urines of such individuals. In secondary hypogonadism, there is definite deficiency of self-produced gonadotropins, and the Leydig cells will respond clinically to the injection of such substances as evidenced by growth of the genitalia. In all cases, testicular biopsy is of great aid in differential diagnosis, for the trend in differential diagnosis, is to depend more and more upon tissue examination, and less on hormone excretion tests. Indeed biopsy of the testis will give information about the physiological potentialities of the impaired testicular function that cannot be obtained by any other test.[2, 4, 5, 6]

In addition bio-assay of urinary androgens are laborious, time-consuming and not always available. What is most significant is that all of the laboratory examinations now available only tell of the amount of androgen excreted, and do not give any informa-

*As a rule the testes in healthy men varies from 1.8 inches to 2 inches in diameter.

tion as to the amount manufactured, and the changes that have occurred to it before it is excreted by the kidneys. In this respect Howard[7] and Scott write: "Colorimetric assay of urinary 17-keto-steroids has been of great value in endocrinological research, but in addition of the criticisms of urinary bio-assay, is subject to still further and greater drawbacks when considered as a poll in the clinical evaluation of male hormone adequacy or deficiency. Depending on the method of extraction used, values of normal adult males vary widely, so that the normal range for the methods must be kept clearly in mind." These authors point out that by one method used, the 24 hour excretion in normal healthy young adults has been found to vary between 20 mg. and 8 mg. and that in the same individual frequently tested, the variation has ranged from 10 to 22 mg. per day with no apparent change in the patient's health or daily routine.

The colorimetric method is the most commonly used test for estimating the total 17-ketosteroids in the urine. As described in chapter five, the term 17-ketosteroids refers to those steroids possessing a ketone group on the 17th carbon atom. It is estimated that a normal male adult excretes up to 27 mg. in the urine per day. Obviously the amounts of 17-ketosteroids found in the urines of males with hypogonadism *will be well below this figure.* Again it must be borne in mind that approximately two-thirds of the androgenic substances found in the urine are of adreno-cortical origin.[8]

But what are these androgens? Androgens are the natural sex hormones and include estrogen, progesterone and androgen which are steroids chemically related to cholesterol and bile acids. The testicular hormone is manufactured by the interstitial cells of Leydig and the hormone is believed to be secreted in the form of testosterone. Without this hormone the male is unable to undergo normal masculine development such as masculine voice, muscular development, masculine hair distribution. In addition it is vital for development and function of the accessory sex glands, as well as for bone growth and closure of the epiphyses. Of singular interest is that these substances are also found in the urine of women, as well as in the urine of children of both sexes.

The internal secretion of the testis, the male sex hormone, is assumed to be elaborated by the interstitial cell of Leydig.[1] This is purely presumptive and has never been proven.[9] However many experiments and clinical observations tend to confirm this belief.[10, 11, 12] The strongest clinical evidence is, as was emphasized in the section on cryptorchidism, adequate androgenic function is maintained where the interstitial cells remain intact despite the fact that the germinal cells undergo destructive and atrophic changes. Masculinity is maintained despite lack of spermatogenesis due to atrophy of germinal cells. In addition the internal secretion is maintained by virtue of the intact Leydig cells which are adequate to stimulate pituitary gonadotropic (ICSH) influence.

As stated above, certain clinical evidence seems to substantiate the belief of a second testicular hormone, but as yet this has not been confirmed.[13, 14, 15] Clinically small amounts of estradiol have been isolated from the human testis.[16] Also following bilateral orchiectomy in man there is a decreased excretion of urinary estrogens.[17] This might however be due to a disturbance of the adreno-cortical testicular balance following the removal of the gonads. Of singular interest is that because of the ability of this hormone to inhibit the pituitary secretion of follicle-stimulating hormone and because of the increased production of FSH following the destruction of the seminiferous tubules (loss of the inhibitory hormone), this hormone has been named by some investigators, "inhibin."

Maddock *et al.*,[19] compared urinary estrogen and 17-ketosteroid excretion with testicular morphology in normal and hypogonadal men, and in men treated with chorionic gonadotropin and luteotrophin, as a means of determining testicular function as well as the true source of estrogen. Estrogen and 17-ketosteroid excretion was extremely low in five cases of hypopituitarism having both testicular and adrenal cortical insufficiency. In seven men lacking only testicular function estrogen excretion was also very low, averaging less than one-fifth normal levels, whereas 17-ketosteroid excretion averaged half that of normal men. The estrogen excretion of two men in whom the only remaining testicular structures were clumps of Leydig cells was definitely greater than castrate levels. These[19] workers then gave chorionic gonadotropin to seven men having functioning testes with a prompt, striking and sustained increase in estrogen excretion, a less marked and more favorable increase in 17 ketosteroid excretion, increased numbers and changes indicative of enhanced secretion of Leydig cells, and regressive changes in the seminiferous tubules. They also noted that when chorionic gonadotropin therapy was given to three hypogonadotropic eunuchoids, growth and development occurred in the Leydig cells, with increase in estrogen excretion from low to several times normal levels and increase in 17 ketosteroids from low to normal levels.

From these observations Maddock[19] and his co-workers concluded: (1) although both the testis and adrenal cortex are important sources of 17 ketosteroids, by far the greater share of urinary estrogens in men originates from the testis; (2) The Leydig cells are the source of testicular estrogens in men; (3) Chorionic gonadotropin stimulates the Leydig cells to secrete both estrogen and androgen; (4) The effects of chorionic gonadotropin are due to its "ICSH actions" rather than its luteotrophin actions, and (5) Urinary estrogen excretion is a more accurate and reliable indicator than 17-ketosteroid determination.

These authors say that "Therefore, the determination of pretreatment urinary estrogen levels and the measurement of changes in estrogen excretion produced by chorionic gonadotropin are suggested as useful procedures for evaluating Leydig cell function."

Androgens are actually transformation products of adrenocortical and testicular steroid hormones, with the greater portion coming from the adrenal cortex. Thus even if laboratory studies reveal normal levels of 17-ketosteroids in the urine of a male this does not necessarily mean the gonadal status is normal in this respect. However when 17-ketosteroids excretion values are elevated in the male with primary hypoadrenocorticism and in young males before puberty, the values are significant. In this respect Talbot[20] and his associates state "Rather surprisingly, in young boys with isosexual precocity due to premature activation of the interstitial cells, the 17-ketosteroid output (±0.3 to 3 mg. per day) is usually only slightly elevated above normal limits for age." This suggests that only a very small amount of testicular androgens are necessary for precocious masculine development or that the gonadal secretion is represented by only a small amount of 17-ketosteroids in the urine. Yet in patients with carcinoma of the interstitial cells of the male gonad, urinary output of 17-ketosteroids is well above normal levels.

The male gonad has two distinct independent functions, i.e., a gametogenic function and a hormonal function. Although theoretically one can assume that either of these functions can be faulty singly or faulty in both functions, it is more practical to assume that hypogametogenesis may exist without gonadal endocrine dysfunction, but one has a strong influence upon the other. Further, a deficiency in one exerts some impairment of the other gonadal function. Of course the age at which such influences occur is significant. For example castration before puberty would result in both gametogenic and endocrine malfunctions. Whereas if late in life (surgical or traumatic) it would result in only gametogenic mal-function and not in endocrine functional disturbances. As stated above failure of the testicle to descend results in failure of *gametogenic* function only. Faulty gametogenic function alone may also be seen in young male adults without any obvious cause.

The significance and role of the hormones in testicular (hypogonadism) physiology cannot be overemphasized.[2,10,21] Thus a defect in spermatogenesis or in the function of the Leydig cells will manifest itself in some hormonal alteration. Gonadotropins will be found in increased amounts in the urine, whenever there is any impairment of the Leydig cells or germ cells. Whenever there is some Leydig cell impairment of function there is found a reduction in the amount of estrogen and androgens in the urine. When the male reaches adult status, the pituitary gland apparently secretes gonadotropins into the blood stream at a constant rate. Failure of the seminiferous tubules and the cells of Leydig to alter the secretions permits assay of urinary gonadotropins as a quantitative laboratory procedure for evaluation of testicular function. In addition circulating androgens and estrogens influence secretion of pituitary gonadotropins in that excess of circulating androgens and estrogens inhibit pituitary secretion of gonadotropins but lack of androgens or estrogens as in testicular failure does not seem to have any effect in increasing gonadotropins. With reduction of gonadotropins due to either (1) excessive estrogens; (2) excessive androgens; or (3) pituitary failure (see below), the Leydig cells regress to mesenchymal cells. Atrophy of the seminiferous tubules soon follows resulting in total testicular atrophy and aspermatogenesis.

Failure of hormonal and germinal functions of the testicles is best illustrated by decrease of the gonadotropic hormones with resultant eunuchism. This entity is characterized physiologically by failure of secretion of the gonadotropic factors (ICSH and FSH) which are absent in the urine. The testes in such cases do not receive the necessary stimulation and morphologically resemble the testes of the pre-adolescent child as to both germinal and secretory components. Hypogonadotropic eunuchoidism actually is an indefinite postponement of puberty. The testes remain small and the seminiferous tubules contain many undifferentiated cells. Few germinal and Sertoli cells are seen with an occasional differentiated spermatogonium. No Leydig cells are seen in the interstitial tissues.

Since there is a definite deficiency of testosterone, the afflicted person suffers from abnormal masculine development. This is characterized by a high pitched voice, little or no hair on the body, face and extremities. The epiphyseal closure is delayed and hence growth continues so that these persons are characterized by tall stature, long arms and legs. There is a characteristic eunuchoid habitus.* Since the adrenal cortex will supply some androgens, untreated hypogonadotropic eunuchoid men will show some pubic and axillary hair at the time of puberty but will not increase thereafter. As stated before, the administration of cho-

---

*The eunuchoid type of skeletal development refers to an abnormal length of the long bones. Clinically this is evaluated by comparison of the lower body measurement (distance from sole to symphysis pubis) with the upper body measurement (distance from symphysis pubis to vertex).

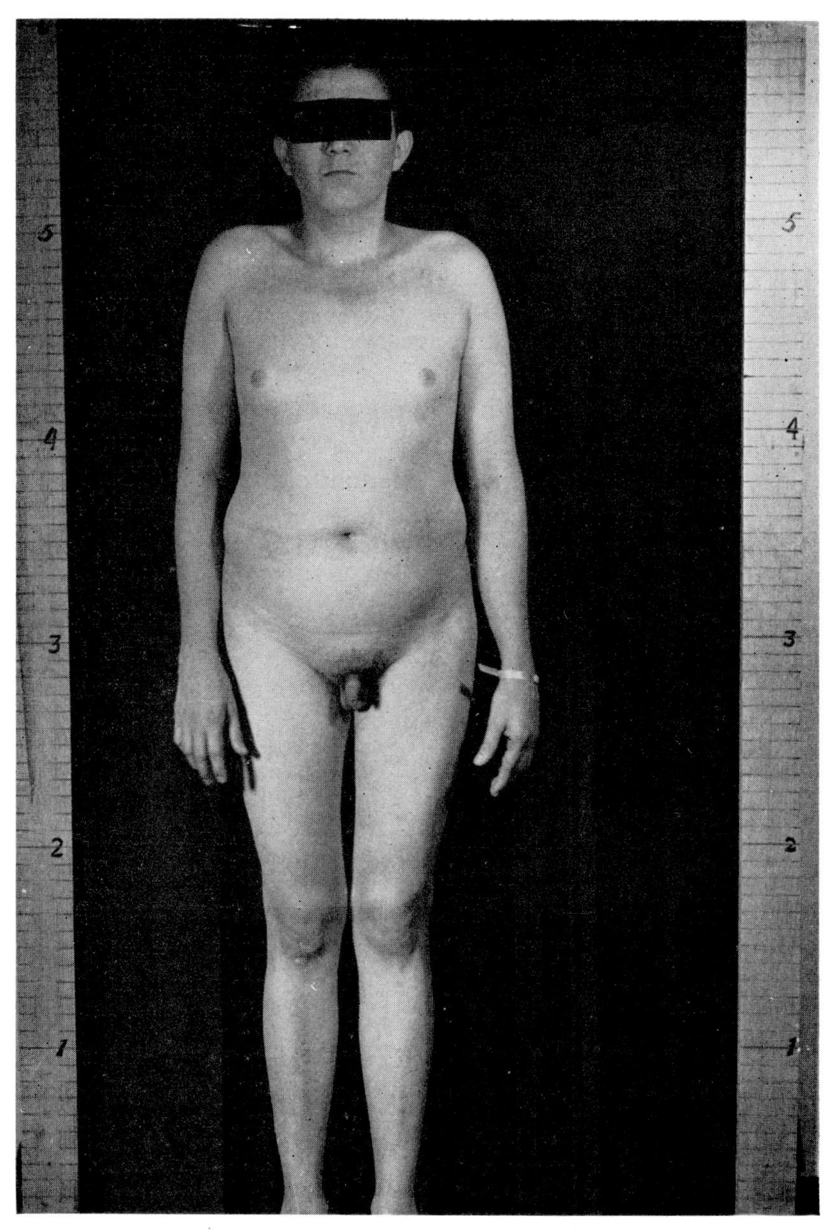

FIG. 17. Eunuchoidism. Aged 59. Note youthful appearance of face, scanty pubic hair and facial hair, length of arms and legs, and small genitalia.

rionic gonadotropin to hypogonadotropic eunuchoid men, accelerates sexual maturation and results in increase in the size of the testes, with increase of estrogen and 17-ketosteroid excretion. Testicular biopsy will reveal increase in the number of interstitial cells of Leydig; enlargement of the seminiferous tubules and Sertoli cells; differentiation of spermatogonia and primary spermato-

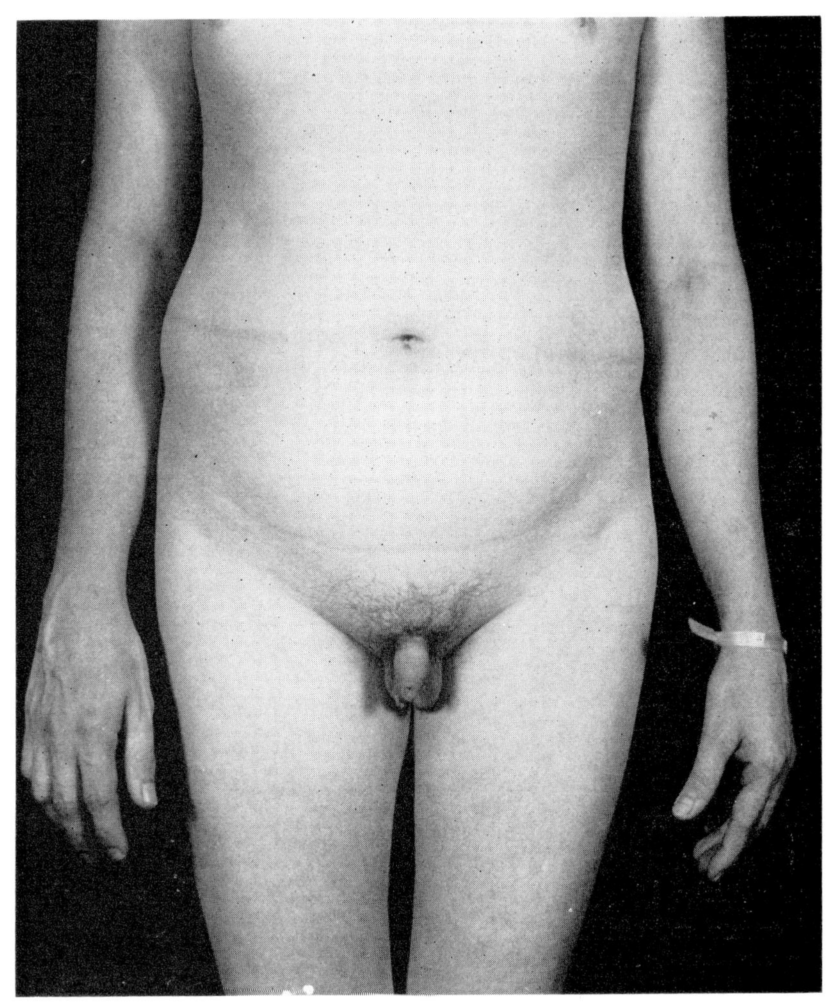

FIG. 18. Close up of genitalia of patient with eunuchoidism (same patient as Figure 17).

cytes. Unfortunately though the germ cells increase in number, their maturation does not proceed to completion.

Eunuchism on the other hand caused by primary failure of the testis, is best spoken of as primary hypogonadism. In this group the time of the gonadal failure is of paramount importance, for if it occurs prior to puberty its manifestations are quite different than if it occurs after puberty and still differ markedly if it occurs later in life. In all cases the cause lies in the testis and is usually accompanied by increase in urinary gonadotropins. The prepuberal eunuch becomes a tall eunuchoid skeleton, sexually infantile and remains so even long after the time of expected puberty. Such cases have failure of both gametogenic and endocrine functions. In contrast the man who is castrated during adult life (surgical, traumatic, inflammatory) does not experience skeletal changes. Secondary sexual changes regress slowly and incompletely and actually may never occur. Some authors believe the most prominent features of adult eunuchoidism are sexual impotence and androgen withdrawal vaso-motor symptoms of the so-called male menopause. This I question.

In the older man, castration has little hormonal effect, as is well demonstrated in those cases subjected to bilateral orchiectomy because of carcinoma of the prostate. In my opinion sex characteristic changes in these males are primarily the result of estrogenic therapy. It is my practice to continue with estrogenic therapy after bilateral orchiectomy, despite the problem of gynecomastia which occurs in most of such cases. This can be controlled by decreasing the dosage of the estrogen or discontinuing it for a day, or administering it on alternate days.

Pituitary eunuchoidism in the male is fairly common in men. The diagnosis is basically made by absence of primary and secondary sexual characteristics, absence of urinary gonadotropins, and a normal prepuberal testicular architecture as obtained by testicular biopsy. Growth may continue for years with resultant eunuchoid habitus.

Obviously absence of a testis (monorchism) or bilateral absence (anorchidism) plays a singular role in the sexual development and maturation of the male. Monorchism should not be

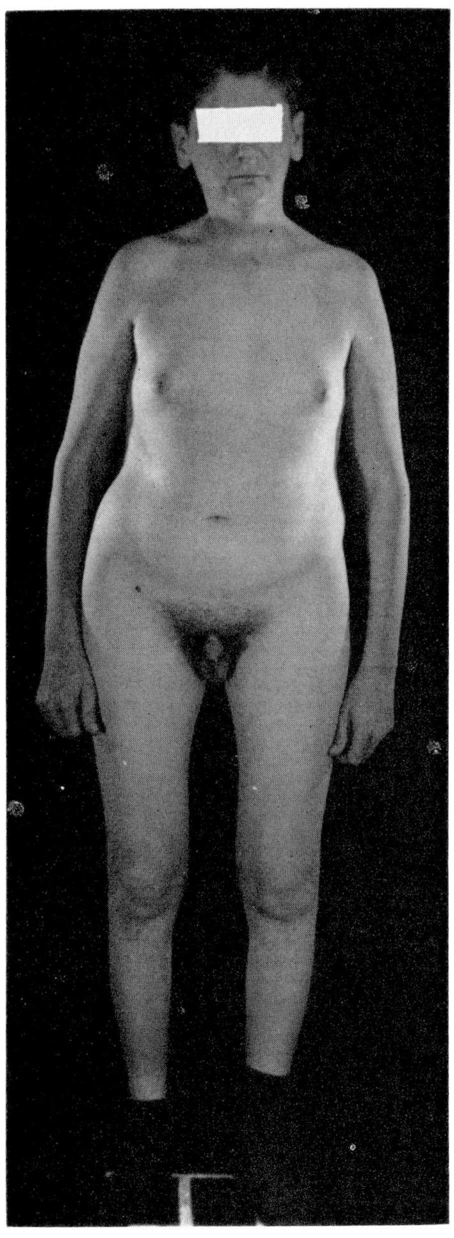

Fig. 19. Eunuchoidism. Age 46. Compare with Figures 17 and 18. These patients closely resemble one another in youthful appearance, scanty facial hair, high pitched voice, long arms and legs and small genitalia.

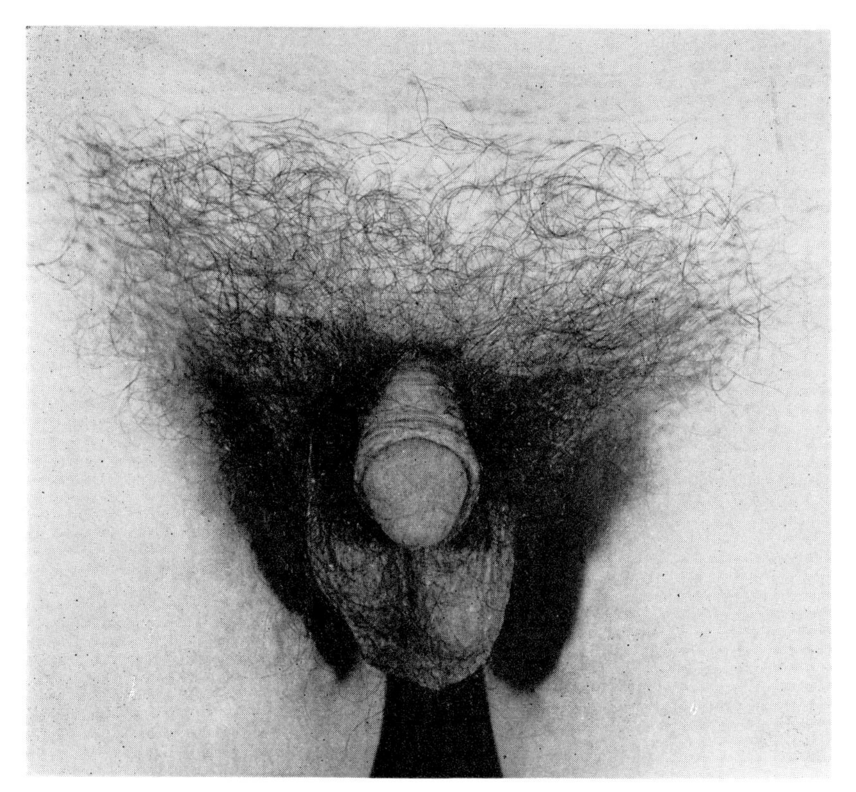

FIG. 20. Close up of genitalia of patient seen in Figure 19. Note feminine distribution of pubic hair.

confused with mal-descent or hypoplasia of the testicle. The diagnosis can only be made when thorough surgical exploration fails to reveal the missing testicle. Clinically it is not as significant as anorchism or congenital absence of both testicles. The author[49] reviewed 14 cases of anorchism found in the literature.

The first case was reported by Cabral,[22] who in 1564 performed an autopsy on a man who had been hanged for rape. No testes were found and it is questionable as to whether the punishment was a just one and whether the man actually performed the crime for which he was hanged. Fisher,[23] in 1839 (this is believed to be the first case reported in America), reports a case of a 45 year old male who died of pneumonia. At no time did this patient have described in 1942 by Klinefelter,[30] Reifenstein and Albright and now spoken of as Klinefelter's syndrome. Despite hypogonadism these patients are entirely masculinized. Ultimately they become sterile. The disorder is characterized by some endocrine dysfunction and definite gametogenic dysfunction.

In 1956, it was first announced that some apparent males with Klinefelter's syndrome had female type nuclei. Since then many cases have been reported and much pertinent information accumulated.[31, 32, 33] Most singular has been the revelation that many of these patients exhibit the female arrangement of their chromosomal pattern.[34, 33, 36] In other words the true sex of these people is subject to debate. The disease is no longer accepted as a rare disease and is now recognized with remarkable frequency. Grumbach[37] believes that the term Klinefelter's syndrome no longer adequately describes this group of patients and he and his associates have proposed the term "seminiferous tubule dysgenesis." This term more adequately indicates a disorder, congenital in nature, and principally evident in the seminiferous tubules.

Klinefelter and his workers emphasize that the disease is usually not recognized prior to puberty as symptoms and signs are not present to this time. This has been disproven by other reports in the literature.[35, 36, 37] The difficulty in clinical diagnosis is apparent when it is realized that few early somatic changes occur during infancy and childhood and that growth and muscular development progresses within normal limits. The testes descend normally and are always in the scrotum. The exernal genitalia are normal in appearance and development. Erections and intercourse are usually satisfactory.

Actually the testes are the first clinical clue to this syndrome. They are usually very small in contrast to the normal genitalia development, measuring about 1½ by ½ cm. The smallness appears on both sides and most patients state that their testes have always been small. Although erections and ejaculations occur azoospermia is present. Reifenstein[38] reports the familiar occurrence of the disorder.

From the above description it can readily be seen that the disease could easily be overlooked in male children before puberty. This is unfortunate for when recognized earlier in life, remedial measures for future fertility could possibly be inaugurated, and as emphasized by workers in this field, even though potential infertility is not of immediate concern in children, appropriate therapy may be instituted early to avoid "the ultimate deforming psychological and anatomical characteristics seen in the adult syndrome."[40] Briggs[39] and his workers advocate chromatin sex determinations as an additional tool in separating the dysgenic endocrinopathies from those due primarily to post natal disturbances in the pituitary gonadal system. These authors point out that the diagnosis can only be made by chromatin sex determinations.

Bunge and Bradbury,[41, 42, 43] report that in an investigation of 8 cases of Klinefelter's syndrome all had positive chromatin tests as seen in normal females and that in further studies in which a gonad from each of three cases were removed, demonstrable histologic evidence of spermatogenesis was present which had not been obtained in biopsy material. These workers believe that the absence of gametogenesis in biopsy specimens from these patients is due to paucity of tubules containing germ cells. In discussing these findings the authors state: "The findings of Klinefelter's syndrome whose gonads show male type germinal cells require an explanation for a paradox. If these patients are genetic males, the chromatin test would be invalid as an index of genetic sex. If these patients are genetic females as indicated by the oral smear or skin biopsy, some causative embryologic deviations must be found to explain the presence of a prostate and scrotal gonads in a female. The lack of beard, the breast development and the female pubic escutcheon are obviously in accord with the female somatic cell findings."

Hamblen[44] in writing on the enigmas in the assignment of sex to an individual speaks of Klinefelter's syndrome as another enigma, in which individuals obviously male, have chromatin positive patterns, gynecomastia, well developed external genitals and scrotal testes, which although small, contain Leydig cells and a degenrated seminiferous tubule epithelium. He refers to Bunge [41, 42, 43] and Bradbury's cases as well as the case of Green and feminine body build with an adipose thorax. Their progress at school was slow. Secondary sex characteristics and gynecomastia were absent in all boys. The nuclear sex, as determined by oral mucosal smears and by skin biopsy in one boy, was "faintly female," the incidence of chromatin positive cells being somewhat lower than in normal females. Such skin biopsy findings are characteristic of Klinefelter's syndrome. In addition to chromatin test and testicular biopsy; the diagnosis of this syndrome is further confirmed by normal or nearly normal development of the masculine secondary sexual characteristics, gynecomastia, abnormally small testes and abnormally elevated urinary FSH output with normal to moderately low urinary 17 ketosteroid excretion.

In a recent study of chromosome pathology in man, Lenz[47] and his co-workers emphasize the improvements in chromosome demonstration, and review recent accomplishments in this field. Thus in the Klinefelter's syndrome, 47 chromosomes are found, and it is assumed that the chromosome complement contains 2 X chromosomes and 1 Y chromosome. These authors stress the theoretical importance of such observations, pointing out that standard concepts of chromosomal sex determination in man must be revised. Attention to increased familial incidence of mongolism and chromatin positive Klinefelter's syndrome must not be overlooked. Also the role of advanced maternal age as a factor predisposing to Klinefelter's syndrome. Two patients in this group had altonism, the male parent had normal color vision but the mothers were heterozygous for the gene for red-green blindness. This was explained through cross-over and nondisjunction in the first miotic division.

Nowakowski[48] and his associates studied 202 patients with primary testicular disease and found 40 to have Klinefelter's syndrome. These authors found clinical symptoms to vary but that hypoplasia of the testes was always present. Their chromatin findings in polymorphonuclear leukocytes differed from those typical in the female, but had to be considered positive. As a further check on the genetic sex, 34 patients were checked for red-green vision, and definite disturbances were found in three. These authors present a hypothesis of etiology in which they believe the syndrome is due to an X chromosome mutation in which the functional, euchromatin-containing segment has been lost, whereas the functionless, heterochromatin-containing part, which is decisive for the chromatin findings, has been spared. They say that "The presence of male gonads can be explained by the fact that only one well-functioning X-chromosome is present. Sterility is due to absence of the Y chromosome."[48]

For sake of completeness, another form of testicular atrophy must be mentioned, namely that seen in myotonia dystrophica. In most clinical reports, the temporal and masseter muscles are atrophic as are the muscles of the hands, of the quadriceps, and the muscles below the knee. Not infrequently (80%), such patients clinically present cataract, impotence, testicular atrophy, baldness, disturbances of speech and loss of the knee jerks.

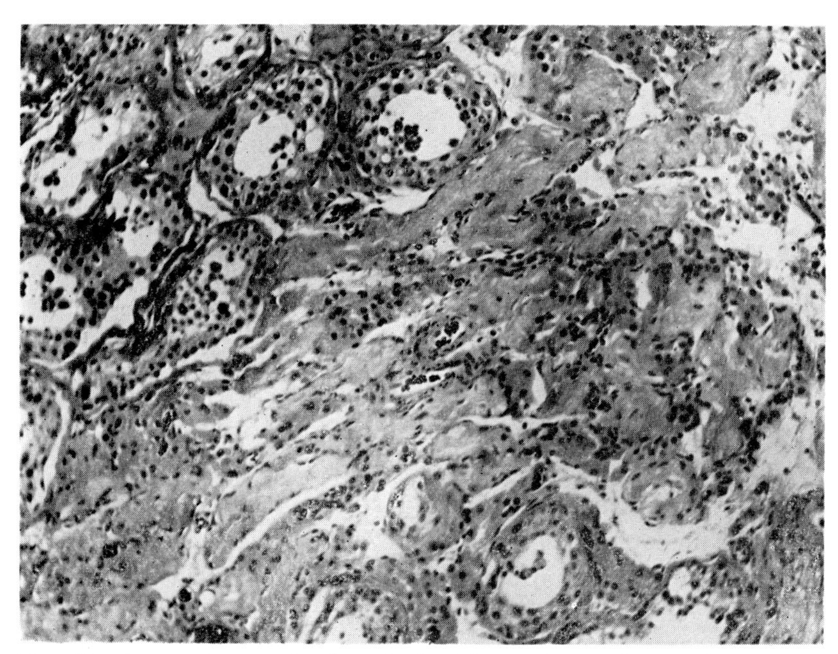

FIG. 23. Photomicrograph of testicular biopsy of a patient with myotonia dystrophica. Note extensive tubular atrophy, diminished spermatogenic elements and few Sertoli cells. Note similarity between this pattern and the pattern of sclerosing tubular degeneration (Klinefelter's syndrome).

The cause of myotonia is a mystery. Clark[50] and his associates have suggested, that since testicular atrophy is associated with myotonia dystrophica as well as other endocrine disorders, this disorder may well represent a concentrated pluriglandular disturbance of endocrine origin. They also offer, "an alternative interpretation in that myotonia atrophica (dystrophia myotonia), rather than reflecting a primary endocrine disturbance, is simply a manifestation of genetically linked degenerative phenomena seen in various tissues derived from embryonic ectoderm and mesoderm."

Of singular interest is the histologic picture of testicular biopsies in these cases. In general the picture is similar to the architectural pattern seen in the testes after mumps, and in adult cryptorchid

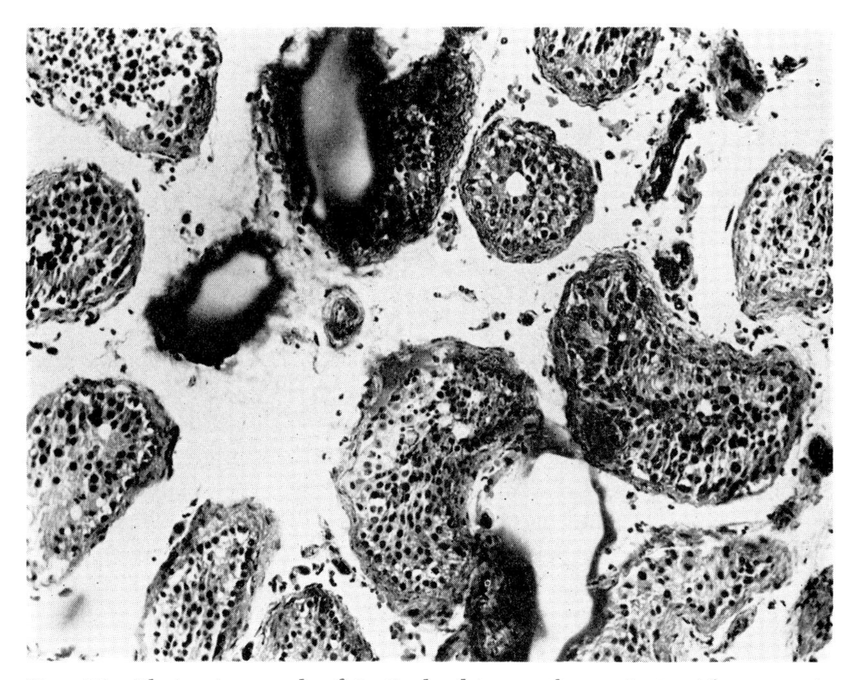

FIG. 24. Photomicrograph of testicular biopsy of a patient with myotonia dystrophica. The tubules are extensively damaged but recognizable as seminiferous. Hyalinization and tubular atrophy is well demonstrated. Again note similarity between this pattern and the pattern of sclerosing tubular degeneration (Klinefelter's syndrome).

testis.[51] Clark *et al.*[60] describe the changes as resembling the testis in Engle's "germinal aplasia." Others[52] describe the changes as similar to those seen in Klinefelter's syndrome. Ledwith[53] and Whipple report a case of myotonia dystrophica with chromatin-negative findings (peripheral smear and skin biopsy). Since many cases of Klinefelter's syndrome are genetic males, Ledwith and Whipple feel that the postulate of Segal and Nelson (mutant gene affects the primordial germ cells) is a plausible explanation. We have recently encountered on the Urologic Service at the Bird S. Coler Hospital several cases of myotonia dystrophica with atrophic testes (clinically). Testicular biopsy demonstrates pathology confined to the seminiferous tubules with extensive tubular atrophy, diminished spermatogenesis, diminished Sertoli cells and intact Leydig's cells (Fig. 23). In one case hyalinization of the seminiferous tubules is well demonstrated (Fig. 24).

REFERENCES

1. Sohval, A. R.: In Soffer's: *Diseases of the Endocrine Glands.* Lea and Febiger, Philadelphia, 2nd edition, p. 470, 1956.
2. Heller, C. G., and Nelson, W. O.: Classification of male hypogonadism. *J. Clin. Endocrinol., 8:* 345-366, 1948.
3. Charney, C. W.: Testicular biopsy; its value in male sterility. *J.A.M.A., 115:* 1429, 1940.
4. Howard, R. P., Simmons, F. A., and Sniffen, R. C.: Differential diagnosis in male sterility. *J. Fertility and Sterility, 2(2):* 95-114, 1951.
5. Sniffen, R. C.: Histology of the normal and abnormal testis at puberty. *Ann. New York Acad. Sc., 55:* 611, 1952.
6. Charney, C. W., Conston, A. S., and Meranze, D. R.: Testicular developmental histology. *Ann. New York Acad. Sc., 55:* 600, 1952.
7. Howard, J. E., and Scott, W. W.: Chapt. 5, The Testes, pp. 316-347. *Textbook of Endocrinology,* 1950.
8. Scott, W. W., and Hudson, P. B.: *Surgery of the Adrenal Glands.* Thomas, Springfield, 1954.
9. Hooker, C. W.: Post natal history and function of the interstitial cells of testis. *Bull. J. Anat., 74:* 1, 1944.
10. Nelson, W. O.: Gamatogenic and endocrine functions of testis. Symposium on Quantitative Biology, Cold Spring Harbor, L. I., N. Y. *The Biological Lab., 5:* 123, 1937.

11. Evans, H. M., Simpson, M. E., and Pencharz, R. I.: An anterior pituitary gonadotropic fraction (ICSH) specifically stimulating the interstitial tissue of testis and ovary. Symposium on Quantitative Biology, Cold Spring Harbor, L. I., N. Y. *The Biological Lab., 5:* 229, 1937.
12. Greep, R. O., Fevold, H. L., and Hisaw, F. L.: Effects of two hypophyseal gonadotropic hormones on reproductive system of male rat. *Anat. Rec., 65:* 261, 1936.
13. Klinefelter, H. F., Jr., Reifenstein, E. C., Jr., and Albright, F.: Syndrome characterized by gynecomastia, aspermatogenesis without A-Leydigism and increased excretion of follicle-stimulating hormone. *J. Clin. Endocrinol., 2:* 615-627, 1942.
14. McCullagh, E. P., Schneider, R. W., Bournam, W., Smith, M. B.: Adrenal and testicular deficiency. *J. Clin. Endocrinol., 8:* 1275, 1948.
15. Howard, R. P. Sniffen, R. C., Simmons, F. A., and Albright, F.: Testicular deficiency. *J. Clin. Endocrinol., 10:* 121, 1950.
16. Goldzieher, J. W., and Roberts, I. S.: Identification of estrogen in the human testis. *J. Clin. Endocrinol. and Metab., 12:* 143, 1952.
17. Kenyon, A. T., Gallagher, T. F., Peterson, D. G., Dorfman, R. I., and Koch, F. C.: Urinary excretion of androgenic and estrogenic substances in certain endocrine states. *J. Clin. Invest., 16:* 705, 1937.
18. McCullagh, D. R.: Dual endocrine activity of testis. Science, *76:* 19, 1932.
19. Maddock, W. O., Epstein, M., and Nelson, W. O.: The assay of urinary estrogens as a test of human leydig cell function. *Ann. New York Acad. of Sc.* Vol. 55, Art. 4, p. 543-742, Nov. 20, 1952.
20. Talbot, N. B., Butler, A. M., and MacLachlan, E. A.: Colorimetric Assay of Total 17-Ketosteroids in Extracts of Human Urine. *J. Biol. Chem.*, 132, 595, 1940.
21. Nelson, W. O.: Testicular morphology in eunuchoidal and infertile men. *J. Fertility and Sterility, 1:* 477-488, 1949.
22. Cabral, B.: Quoted by Hepburn, R. H. Anorchism. *J. Urol., 62:* 65, 1949.
23. Fisher, N.: Quoted by Hepburn, R. H. Anorchism. *J. Urol., 62:* 65, 1949.
24. Godard, A. B.: Quoted by Hepburn, R. H. Anorchism. *J. Urol., 62:* 65, 1949.
25. Wieldboltz, H.: Ein Fall von Kongenitaler Anorchie. Cor. *Bl. of Schweiz. Aerzte., 47:* 1307, 1917.
26. Koopman, J.: Anorchia Congenita. *Genesk. gids, 8:* 309, 1930.
27. Counseller, U. S., and Walker, M. S.: Congenital absence of testes. *Am. Surg., 98:* 104-109, 1933.
28. Hepburn, R. H.: Anorchism. *J. Urol., 62:* 65, 1949.
29. Amelar, R. D.: Anorchism without eunuchism. *J. Urol., 76:* 174, 1956.

30. Klinefelter, H. F., Reifenstein, E. C., and Albright, F.: Syndrome characterized by gynecomastia, aspermatogenesis without A-Leydigism and increased excretion of follicle-stimulating hormone. *J. Clin. Endocrinol, 2:* 615, 1942.
31. Nelson, W. O., and Heller, C. G.: Hyalinazation of Seminiferous tubules associated with normal or failing Leydig cell function. *J. Clin. Endocrinol., 5:* 13, 1945.
32. Sniffen, R. C., Howard, R. P., and Simmons, F. A.: The Testis III. Absence of germ cells; sclerosing tubular degeneration; "Male Climacteric." *Arch. Path., 51:* 293, 1951.
33. Davidson, W. M., and Smith, R. D.: *The Neutrophil Sex Nodules in Klinefelter's Syndrome: Symposium on Nuclear Sex.* p. 93. William Heinmann Medical Books, LTD, London.
34. Wildemann, H. R.: *The Result of Hematological Determination of the Genetic Sex in Disturbances of Sexual Development; Symposium on Nuclear Sex,* p. 14, William Heinmann Medical Books, LTD., London.
35. Lennox, B., Ferguson-Smith, M. A., Mack, W. S., and Stewart, J. S. S.: *Frequency of Klinefelter's Syndrome and the Relationships of Chromatin-Positive and Chromatin-Negative Cases; Symposium on Nuclear Sex,* p. 112, William Heinemann Medical Books, LTD, London.
36. Siebenman, R. E.: *Gonadal Histology and Nuclear Morphology in Klinefelter's Syndrome.* William Heinemann Medical Books, LTD, p. 116, London.
37. Grumbach, M. M.: Special Article: The sex chromatin pattern and human sexual anomalies. *Year Book of Endocrinology,* 1958-1959. Year Book Publishers, Chicago, p. 281.
38. Reifenstein, E. C., Jr.: Quoted by Grumbach, M. M., Van Wyck, J. J., and Wilkins, L. J. *Clin. Endocrinol., 15:* 116, 1955.
39. Briggs, D. K., Epstein, J., and Kupperman, H. S.: The place of chromatin sex determinations in Klinefelter's syndrome. *J. Urol.,* 80, 57, 1958.
40. Briggs, D. K., Epstein, J., and Kupperman, H. S.: The place of chromatin sex determinations in Klinefelter's syndrome. *J. Urol.,* Vol. 80, July, 1958, p. 57.
41. Bunge, R. G., and Bradbury, J. T.: Hermaphrod., Pseudo. *J. Urol., 77:* 759, 1957.
42. Bunge, R. G., and Bradbury, J. T.: Newer concepts of the Klinefelter's syndrome. *J. Urol., 76:* 758, 1956.
43. Bunge, R. G., and Bradbury, J. T.: A 10-Year-Old Boy with a Positive Sex Chromatin Test. *J. Urol., 76:* 775, 1957.
44. Hamblen, E. C.: The assignment of sex to an individual; some enigmas and some practical clinical criteria. *Am. J. Obst. and Gynec., 74:* 1228-1244, 1957.

45. Witchi, E., Nelson, W. O., and Segal, S. J.: Genetic, developmental and hormonal aspects of gonadal dysgenesis and sex inversion in man. *J. Clin. Endocrinol., 17:* 737, 1957.
46. Siebenmann and Prader, A.: The Klinefelter syndrome before puberty. *Schweiz. Med. Wchnschr., 88:* 607-6110, June 21, 1958.
47. Lenz, W., Nowakowski, H., Prader, A., and Schirren, G.: Etiology of the Klinefelter syndrome; Contribution to chromosome pathology in man. *Schweiz. Med. Wchnschr., 89:* 727-731, July 11, 1958.
48. Nowakowski, H., Lenz., W., and Prada, J.: Discrepancy between chromatin findings and genetic sex in Klinefelter's syndrome. *Acta Endocrinol., 30:* 296-320, Feb. 1959.
49. Wershub, L. P.: *Sexual Impotence in the Male.* Thomas, Springfield, 1959.
50. Clark, B. G., Shapiro, S., Monroe, R. G.: Myotonia atrophica with testicular atrophy: urinary excretion of interstitial cell-stimulating (lutenizing) hormone, androgens and 17-ketosteroids. *J. Clin. Endocrin., 16:* 1235, 1956.
51. Sohval, A. R., and Soffer, L. J.: Congenital familial testicular deficiency. *Am. J. Med., 14:* 328, 1953.
52. Jacobson, W. E., Schultz, A. L., and Anderson, J.: Endocrine studies in eight patients with dystrophia myotonica. *J. Clin. Endocrinol., 15:* 801, 1955.
53. Ledwith, J. W., and Whipple, R. J.: Myotonia Dystrophica: A case report with sex chromatin studies. *Annals Int. Med., 54:* 113, 1961.

Chapter 11

THE TESTES AND THE ADRENALS

IN 1955, HIGGINS[1] wrote a classic review of the great advances made in urology from 1905 to 1955. In it he spoke of the great strides made in adrenal physiology, pathology and adrenal surgery. "Currently, these glands, their physiology, hormones, biochemistry and pathology, offer one of the most active fields for experimental and clinical research not only with regard to urology but to all other departments of medicine and surgery. As knowledge has accumulated concerning the functions and dysfunctions of the adrenal glands, steady progress has been made in the diagnosis of adrenal disease and its treatment. As more and more has been learned about the physiologic effects of the cortical hormones, a clearer conception has been gained of their complexity. More research still remains to be done in the future to elucidate completely the function of these tiny glands which are indispensible to health and life. Although it is impossible to predict where the next discovery relating to the adrenal glands may lead, present studies apparently are aiming toward clearer concepts of the role of the adrenocortical hormones in relation to electrolytic balance, metabolism of the carbohydrates and fats, and to certain sexual abnormalities, such as virilism and pseudohermaphroditism."

Higgins wrote his review in 1955 and since then many tests of adrenal dysfunction are now routine in clinical hormonal investigations. The relationship of the adrenal with the testis is most obvious, yet clinically it is confusing. A clear, concise understanding of this interrelationship is essential for successful recognition and therapy. This will be stressed in this chapter.

Since embryologically, the male gonad[2,3,4,5,6,7] and the adrenal cortices arise from adjacent structures, it is not unusual that cells which are histologically identical with adrenal cortical cells, are occasionally found in the body of the testis. That the testes and adrenal cortex should form identical steroids is also not surprising when one considers their common embryologic ancestry. Not only are these steroids similar in chemical structure but they are also quite similiar in physiological action.

The hormonal influence of the adrenal cortex, on life preservation, is not as yet entirely understood. However the action of its secretions can be divided into three separate categories;[8] (1) those which influence the metabolism of body fluids and electrolytes; (2) those which act on sugar, fat and protein metabolism; and (3) those which influence sex, hair growth, and acne. The actions of (1) and (2) are usually referred to as "*corticoid*" and (3) as "*androgenic,*" "*estrogenic*" and "*progestational.*" Under abnormal conditions the adrenal cortex may secrete appreciable amounts of androgens, estrogens and other types of hormones. The cells arranged in three zones (glomerulosa, fasciculata and reticularis) are believed by some to be concerned with the specific secretion of (1) electrolyte-regulating; (2) glucogenetic; and (3) androgenic hormones. However this has never been proven and it is more likely that other alternatives are possible. This theory at times has given rise to the popular belief that the adrenal cortex is actually three organs in one, each with a special function.

Androgenic Hormones: The adrenal cortices normally commence to produce urinary 17-ketosteroids between the eighth and tenth years of life.[9, 10, 11] As a rule there is a close parallelism between the biologic androgenic manifestations seen in a patient and the level of 17-ketosteroids excreted. *The 17-ketosteroids are derived from both adrenal and testicular steroids having the chemical configuration of androgens.* A small amount (5%) of adrenal corticosteroids may be metabolized to 17-ketosteroids. In adrenal disorders the level of urinary 17-ketosteroids may be used as a rough index of the androgenic activity of the adrenals. The adrenocortical androgens have a weak androgenic action and do not cause development of the penis in the male or of the clitoris in the female. They do stimulate pubic and axillary hair and are capable of producing acne. Deficiency of these hormones is clinically of little importance. When present in excessive amounts clinical disturbances become obvious. This is seen in adrenogenital virilism with bilateral adrenal hyperplasia or with adrenal tumor.

HYPERFUNCTION OF THE ADRENAL CORTEX

Hyperfunction of the adrenal cortex may manifest itself as either: (1) the adrenogenital syndrome; (2) Cushing's syndrome; (3) primary aldosteronism; or (4) feminizing adrenal tumors in males. The specific form is entirely dependent upon which of the cortical cells will secrete an excess of one or all of the different type of adrenal cortical secretions. Thus if androgens predominate or there is an excess of hydro-cortisone-like substances, *the adrenogenital syndrome* manifests itself. This may be the result of either bilateral hyperplasia of the adrenals or an adrenal tumor. If as in the presence of an adenoma or carcinoma and hyperplasia there is an excess in secretion, and hydrocortisone and cortisone like substances predominate, *Cushing's syndrome* manifests itself. When the secretions contain an excess of aldosterone, *Primary aldosteronism* results, and finally, *feminizing adrenal tumors* in males occurs with estrogenic tumors of the adrenal cortex.

Much confusion and misleading clinical interpretation exists about diseases classified by most endocrinologists under the headings of "virilism," "Cushing's Syndrome" and the "adrenogenital syndrome." I quite agree with Soffer[9] who believes that the reasons for the confusion, "resides in part in the apparently large numbers of etiologic factors with which the clinical picture has been associated and in part because of the variety of clinical manifestations that the disease, or perhaps diseases, has assumed." Thus since four varieties of steroids are produced by the adrenal cortex: (1) androgens; (2) glucocorticoids (cortisone); (3) mineralocorticoids (aldosterone); and 4) estrogen, it follows that different symptoms and different clinical manifestations may occur as a result of excessive secretion of a specific adrenocortical steroid.

Since we are primarily interested in the testes, and the signs and symptoms associated with sexual abnormalities, we will confine our discussion to the mechanism of the so-called adrenogenital syndrome. As an aid in differential diagnosis and because of clinical overlapping, reference to Cushing's syndrome will be made. For sake of completeness a short discussion of aldosterone in man, will be included in this chapter. For a more detailed description of hyperfunction of the adrenal cortex, the reader is referred to any standard text book on endocrinology.[9, 10, 11]

Adreno-genital Syndrome: The adreno-genital syndrome is a clinical entity characterized by disturbances and changes in the structure and function of the genitals accompanied by excessive metabolic activity. The recognition of this syndrome and the value of hormonal therapy is receiving more and more attention from urologists. The disease is a typical example of an inborn error of hormonal metabolism in man.

Obviously the clinical picture of the adreno-genital syndrome varies according to the age of the patient at the time of hyperfunction of the adrenals and of course according to the sex of the afflicted person. For simplication it is well to divide cases of adrenogenital syndrome into: (a) Pre-natal, resulting in pseudohermaphroditism in the female and macrogenitosomia praecox in the male; (b) Prepuberal, resulting in virilization in the female and precocious pseudo-sexual development in the male; (c) Adult, with signs of virilization in the female and excessive sexual development in the male.

a. Pre-natal disturbances: Such a disturbance is the direct result of hypersecretion of the adrenal cortex. This may be due to hyperplasia or tumor of the adrenal cortex. It may also exist without any gross or microscopic changes in the adrenal cortex. When the fetus is a female, marked signs of masculinization occurs. At birth such a female will have marked enlargement of the clitoris with malformation of the external genitalia. This is the clinical entity spoken of as pseudohermaphroditism. The diagnosis is based upon the clinical findings and elevated urinary 17-ketosteroids.

Differential diagnosis is essential for the disorder may be due to either bilateral cortical hyperplasia, or cortical tumor (benign or malignant). A positive diagnosis can only be made by direct surgical exposure of the adrenal glands. This may be difficult or even impossible since surgery is not always an elective procedure. As a rule patients exhibiting (especially in the female) congenital defects of the lower genital tract usually have adrenocortical hyperplasia rathen then neoplasia. Patients with bilateral cortical hyperplasia can be inhibited in their production of ACTH by the administration of cortisone. This does not occur with adrenocortical tumor and there is no significant decrease in the production of urinary 17-ketosteroids despite the administration of cortisone.

In female pseudohermaphroditism a variety of malformations of the external genitalia are seen shortly after birth. Most workers stress the importance of early diagnosis especially in infancy as a means of preventing unhappy adult development and later serious inter-sex problems. The clitoris is often so enlarged as to be frequently mistaken for a penis. The hypertrophied clitoris closely resembles a hypospadic penis bound ventrally in a position of chordee with marked variations in the degree of fusion of the labioscrotal folds. No gonads are palpable within the fused genital folds which often has given the physician the erroneous impression of *male cryptorchidism* when in reality the child is a *female pseudohermaphrodite*. At times there is no fusion and the vulva appears normal in outline with separate urethral and vaginal openings. Wilkins[12] describes cases where the labioscrotal folds extends anteriorly nearly to the base of the phallus. "This results in the formation of a scrotal-like structure with a median raphe and the conversion of the urogenital sulcus into a tube opening into a slit or a small meatus situated at the base of the phallus. Urethroscopic examination of the urogenital sinus usually reveals the communication with the vagina and the cervix of the uterus can often be visualized." Otherwise the sex differentiation is entirely female.

Such children grow rapidly and for a time are above the average weight and height (early adolescent epiphyseal closure). Full growth may be reached by 10 years of age, so that as adults they are usually shorter than the normal adult. As in other forms of the adreno-genital syndrome, these children will show clinical signs of virilization with early appearance of pubic hair followed by distribution of axillary hair and body hair. In some cases the

The urine was normal. The excretion levels of 17-ketosteroids and 11-hydroxysteroids were 0.4 and 1.5 mg. per twenty-four hours, respectfully. The excretion of pituitary gonadotropins was 11 rat units (normal adult level, 5-10 rat units) per twenty-four hours. A toad test for chorionic gonadtropins was negative.

An intravenous pyelogram and abdominal films demonstrated an irregular calcific density anterior to the kidney in the right upper quadrant of the abdomen; a spina bifida was observed at the level of the third sacral vertebra; the contrast media was excreted promptly and in good concentration bilaterally; the calyceal patterns were normal.

A testicular biopsy specimen revealed Leydig-cell hyperplasia and slight tubular enlargement; there was no evidence of spermatogenesis. The striking development of large, polyhedral Leydig cells in contrast to an interstitium composed almost entirely of collagenous tissue as seen in the normal testis, at this age, was quite striking.

At exploration a large friable, necrotic tumor was found, arising in the right lobe of the liver and extending into the left lobe. It was inoperable. Biopsy revealed it to be a hepatoma. The virilism increased as the tumor enlarged, and the hemoglobin and platelet levels fell. Patient expired three months after the exploration. At autopsy, a large mass was found occupying the major part of the right lobe and extending into the left lobe. Microscopically, the tumor was composed of cords of cells separated by sinusoidal spaces lined by endothelium—typical architecture of a primary liver-cell carcinoma, or hepatoma.

c. Adult Disturbances: The adreno-genital syndrome is not too rare a disease among adults where the disturbance is the result of hypersecretion of androgenic adrenal hormones. In the adult female, the masculinization is not as marked as when the hypersecretion occurs before puberty or during the pre-natal phase. Such women exhibit hirsuitism (most marked on face, trunk and limbs), arrest of ovarian function with disturbed menses and inability to conceive. In most instances the *primary dysfunction is due to adrenal tumor* but the cause is sometimes traced to adrenocortical hyperplasia. At times the diagnosis can only be made by surgical exploration and at times even then the diagnosis cannot be confirmed despite careful histologic study of section taken at exploration. When the tumor is present (usually carcinoma) the diagnosis is made on the following data: (1) *masculinization not marked and only of recent date;* (2) *definite displacement of kidney on involved side;* (3) *marked elevation of total urinary 17-ketosteroids;* (4) *normal blood chemistry;* (5) *no metabolic disturbances suggestive of Cushing's syndrome.*

The adreno-genital syndrome is more prevalent among women than men.[35] In the adult male hypersecretion of the adrenal cortex, due to a cortical tumor may result in the so-called feminizing tumor of the adrenal cortex. As a rule hyperfunction of the adrenal cortex caused by a tumor gives the clinical picture described in Cushing's syndrome. However hyperfunction caused by a tumor may manifest itself in an entirely different manner—namely feminization. Higgins,[35] Brownlee and Mantz have reviewed only 27 cases of feminizing adrenal cortical tumors in males. Wallach,[36] Brown, Enlert and Eiknes report the occurrence of a feminizing adrenocortical carcinoma in a patient whose presenting complaint was gynecomastia. It is of singular interest to note that Wallach et al found 33 cases of feminizing adrenal cortical tumor in the literature to October, 1956, and add their own case, making the total to this date of 34 cases of feminizing adrenal cortical tumors reported in the literature.

The case reported by Wallach[36] and his associates is of interest and reads as follows:

> Man, 28, had intermittently tender nipples and later, bilateral breast enlargement and gradual decline in libido and potency. No fluctuations in weight were observed. Physical examination revealed pubic and axillary hair in moderate amounts, the former of feminine distribution. The beard was sparse. The breasts were considerably enlarged, with palpable sub-areolar glandular tissue, deeply pigmented, nontender nipples and prominent Montgomery tubules. The testes measured 1.5 to 2 cm. in diameter and were smooth and firm. The penis and prostate were normal. Laboratory studies revealed elevated urinary excretion of estrogen, normal excretion of 17-ketosteroids, absence of chorionic gonadotropin and follicle-

stimulating hormone in the urine, a fat glucose tolerance curve and a response to ACTH that was indicative of relative adreno-cortical insufficiency. Surgery revealed a large solid tumor occupying the right adrenal area. Microscopically the specimen revealed cortical carcinoma of the right adrenal gland. Of interest post-operatively is that though the breasts were slightly prominent, no glandular tissue was palpable, 12 months after surgery. Pulmonary metastases developed 2 years after excision.

In all cases, *gynecomastia* has been an outstanding sign and for this reason the author wishes to emphasize this sign but equally warn the reader that breast enlargement is not necessarily a sign of feminizing adreno-cortical tumor in the male. It is especially well to distinguish gynecomastia of adolescent males. In this respect Wilkins[17] states: "Breast enlargement, which may be either unilateral or bilateral, frequently occurs in adolescent boys who are otherwise apparently normal. It is particularly apt to occur in boys who are virilizing rapidly. The condition is often slight and transitory but at times the breast may attain considerable size and persist for many years. The cause of gynecomastia during adolescence is not known. It is possible that estrogens are secreted in excess by the adrenals or testes or that there is a temporary disproportion in different types of testicular hormones." Wilkins[16] claims adolescent gynecomastia can be differentiated from that which occurs in Klinefelter's syndrome by the fact that the testes are of *normal adolescent or adult size.* In Klinefelter's syndrome the *testes are small* and azoospermia is present.

In a review of the tabulations of cases of feminizing tumors of the adrenal cortex reported in the literature one is impressed with: (1) breast change *(gynecomastia)* is the most constant symptom and is present in the majority of the recorded cases. In many instances the breast resemble those of a well developed female of the same age. It is of interest to note that breast enlargement may be delayed, slow and often developing to a marked degree in one breast before the other; (2) *feminizing hair* changes are not as prevalent as gynecomastia but when present is characterized by a feminine distribution of the supra-pubic hair and a thinning of the beard; (3) *atrophic* changes of the testes occurs and this is usually bilateral; (4) although the size of the penis has been described as smaller than normal in some cases, this does not seem to be a reasonable finding; (5) in a small percentage of cases there appears some increase in pigmentation of the skin and acne in an even smaller group of cases; (6) pain at the site of the tumor is a late symptom and when it does occur is usually associated with adrenal cortical carcinoma rather than adrenal cortical adenoma; and (7) diminished or absent libido accompanied by a decrease or loss of potency may occur either early in the disease or at a more gradual and progressive rate as compared to the growth of the cortical tumor.

It follows that the diagnosis of a feminizing tumor of the adrenal cortex can be made from the history, the physical examination, x-ray demonstration of a supra-adrenal mass by either retrograde pyelograms, the latter best done in conjunction with the retroperitoneal air insufflation, as well as laboratory evidence of increased urinary excretion of corticosteroid products. In this respect it is well to remember that as a rule the 17-ketosteroids are increased in the urine in cases of adrenal cortical carcinoma. The number of reported cases of feminizing tumors of the adrenal cortex is small and no good corollary has been made in this respect. However it appears safe to assume from the number of cases reported in the literature that large quantities of 17-ketosteroids are excreted in the urine by feminizing tumors of the adrenal cortex.

CUSHING'S SYNDROME

For sake of completeness, the author has included Cushing's syndrome. There is no simple or single rule whereby it is possible to determine whether an adrenal tumor or hyperplasia is the underlying cause of this syndrome. The actual diagnosis can only be confirmed by surgical exploration. Indeed in all cases of suspected Cushing's syndrome exploration of both adrenals is advised, for if due to neoplasia, surgical excision offers the chance for cure.

In 1932, Harvey Cushing reported a group of patients with a clinical picture and distinctive symptoms which has since been spoken of as Cushing's syndrome. The term Cushing's disease was formerly used for cases of bilateral adrenal cortical hyperplasia associated with a demonstrable basophilic adenoma, whereas today it is applied to the clinical picture which though identical may occur as a result of (a) tumor of the cortex of the adrenal gland; (b) bilateral hyperplasia of the adrenal cortex; or (c) normal adrenal cortex with tumor of the anterior lobe of the hypophysis. Cushing's original description of the clinical picture still holds good today.

The clinical picture is classical. It is characterized by the following: (1) obese individuals with centripetal fat distribution especially marked in the supra clavicular regions, on the back of the neck (buffalo hump) and in the face (moonface and fish mouth), yet characteristically sparing the extremities; (2) the skin has lost its elasticity, has wide striae of purplish hue, heals poorly, easily bruised and usually in addition to the purplish striae exhibits numerous areas of ecchymosis; (3) marked osteoporesis with dorsal kyphosis and ultimate compression fractures of the vertebrae; (4) hyperglycemia and glycosuria; (5) hypertension; (6) sexual impotence in the male; and (7) hirsuitism and amenorrhea in the female.

The reader must bear in mind that all these symptoms and signs may not be present early in the disease and many of the so called classic signs of the disease may be entirely absent. The affliction is more common in women than in men (5-1).

Roentgenograms are of aid in detecting Cushing's syndrome but here too it must be emphasized that there is no roentgen change which in itself is pathognomonic of Cushing's syndrome. However the following should arouse suspicion of the disease: (1) osteoporesis when present seems to be confined to the skull, rib, spine and pelvis with sparing of the extremities; (2) bone age in young patients is most often retarded; and (3) the so-called "bolded" rib fractures are common and usually spontaneous in onset.

Hinman[37] and his associates believe that a rounder or oval mass seen on pneumograms is virtually diagnostic of adrenal neoplasm if corticoid excretion is elevated. They also believe that a large triangular adrenal associated with contralateral atrophy is also indicative of tumor. A small adrenal should arouse suspicion of neoplasm on the opposite side. An adenoma appears symmetrical, whereas a carcinoma appears irregular. The value of extraperitoneal pneumography is usually enhanced by simultaneous pyelography.

Laboratory studies reveal polycythemia, with elevated hemoglobin and hematocrit. Eosinopenia is usually if not always present. Urinalysis may be entirely normal if not complicated by diabetes mellitus or hypertension. Frequently seen is the trend toward extra-cellular alkalosis, with elevation of the serum chlorides and potassium. It is believed that these changes are the result of intracellular acidosis resulting from the exchange of two sodium ions and a hydrogen ion for three potassium ions produced by excess cortico steroid secretion.

The diagnosis is made on the demonstration of hyperfunction of the adrenal cortex. Thus an elevation in the urinary output (24 hours) of 17-ketosteroids above 12 mg. is highly suggestive of Cushing's syndrome, provided the patient is not under stress, has no liver damage and is not taking ACTH or cortisone. Here it must be emphasized that the determination of the 24 hour urinary excretion of 17-Ketosteroids is not in itself adequate. A more accurate test is to include determination of the more important 17-hydroxycorticoids in order to distinguish (if possible) between Cushing's syndrome and the adrenogenital syndrome. In Cushing's syndrome the 17-ketosteroids rarely go above 15 mg. per day in the female and 20 mg. per day in the male (expressed as dehydroepiandrosterone equivalents) except in the presence of carcinoma, whereas in the adrenogenital syndrome levels of 30 mg. per day or even higher are found.

ALDOSTERONISM

Aldosteronism in man is now accepted as an important clinical entity. As evidence is accumulated the disorder appears to have significant influence in the regulation of electrolyte balance and arterial pressure by a specific renal and adrenal system.

Subsequent to the demonstration of the remarkable and unparalleled biological effects of hydrocortisone, most investigators were willing to recognize this steroid (hydrocortisone) as the major and toti-potent hormone secreted by the adrenal cortex.[38]

In 1950, Deming[39] and Luetscher reported that steroidal extracts of urine from patients forming edema contained a material which was potent in promoting sodium retention and potassium excretion in adrenalectomized rats. This was followed by the isolation and characterization of the adrenal cortical hormone *aldosterone*.[40]

Although aldosterone is present in extremely minute amounts in plasma (one one-hundredth of the concentration of hydrocortisone) it is extremely potent in that it appears to play a significant role in the regulation of potassium and sodium in the body. Of significant interest is that its direct action in the renal tubule is to accelerate renal retention of sodium chloride and to eliminate potassium crisis.

It has been shown that the adrenal cortex of normal subjects secrete about 250 meg. per day. When sodium is lacking the secretory rate may rise to levels of 1,000 meg. per day and with administration of sodium chloride the level falls to 50 meg. per day.[41] "From a practical point of view this means that one must always take into account the state of salt and water balance in determining the significance of an aldosterone measurement."[41]

Unlike hydrocortisone, aldosterone has very little anti-inflammatory activity. It also differs from cortisone in that its rate of secretion is not regulated primarily by ACTH (the rate of secretions of hydrocortisone is regulated by the amount of ACTH, its trophic hormone, that is secreted by the anterior pituitary, the blood level of hydro-cortisone, which results from ACTH stimulation, acts in turn to suppress further productions of ACTH). Thus the adrenal cortex is the source of at least two different hormones with different controlling systems and with different purposes.[42]

Excessive aldosterone excretion can occur from functional hyperplasia of the adrenal cortex.[43] Unfortunately this cannot be detected by simple palpation at exploration. Fortunately because of the availability of potent steroid preparations, adrenalectomy may now be performed when the clinical and laboratory picture of aldosteronism warrants such a procedure, even though the gross picture is not exclusive. Only about one-third of small aldosterone-producing tumors can be demonstrated by roentgen examination (gas insufflation).[44]

Primary aldosteronism is characterized by excessive amounts of sodium-retaining corticoid in the urine, severe hypokalemia, hypernatremia, alkalosis and a renal tubular defect in the reabsorption of water. These cases are identified by intermittent tetany, paresthesia, periodic severe muscular weakness and "paralysis," polyuria, polydipsia, hypertension but no edema.

Delorme[44] and Genest emphasize that the plasma potassium determinations are indicated in every hypertensive case, regardless of age. Hypokalemia is a constant finding in all cases, with alkalosis present in most cases, varying from a slight to a marked degree. These authors also stress that urinary aldosterone is elevated in most cases; with a large urinary loss of potassium; but that urinary 17-hydrocortico steroids and 17-ketosteroids excretions are normal.

Thus when hypersecretion of aldosterone develops in an individual, the syndrome of primary aldosteronism develops characterized by (1) arterial hypertension; (2) potassium wastage with associated hypokalemic alkalosis; (3) muscle weakness; and (4) polyuria. Such symptoms are all reversed if due to adenoma when removed by adrenalectomy. As a matter of fact surgery is the only definitive form of treatment.

There is no doubt that increasing number of cases of aldosteronism will be detected and that many will require surgical exploration. Since some will have benign cortical adenomas and others no demonstrable lesion the decision for surgery becomes complicated. Its indication can however not be denied even though the differential diagnosis still remains difficult.

SUMMARY

Adrenal cortical hyperfunction producing sexual abnormalities can be divided into two large groups.[9] *The first group* includes the female with signs of virilism, and include hirsuitism, enlargement of the clitoris, development of male musculature, deepening of the voice, acne and amenorrhea. In the prepuberal male the sexual abnormalities include isosexual precocity. In the post puberal male feminization may occur.

The second group includes those patients with signs and symptoms associated with metabolic disturbances namely: "Cushing's syndrome." The reader must bear in mind that a typical clinical picture of this syndrome may be present, without any glandular pathology. Cushing's syndrome may be encountered with a basophilic adenoma, adrenocortical hyperplasia and adrenal tumor, benign or malignant. In addition basophilic adenomas of the pituitary and adrenal cortical tumors have been found in patients without symptoms of virilism or symptoms of Cushing's syndrome. Finally most of the symptoms of the disease whether true adrenogenital syndrome or Cushing's syndrome, are due to a disturbance of the adrenal cortical function.

Diagnosis of congenital virilizing adrenal hyperplasia is based on signs of *virilization, elevated 17-ketosteroid* excretion and suppressibilty of 17-ketosteroid levels with hydrocortisone like steroids.[46] Suppression of 17-ketosteroids does not occur with adrenal tumor.[47] In true precocious puberty, the 17-ketosteroids are normal when related to the patient's bone age, though elevated in regard to the chronologic age. Further, virilizing adrenal and gonadal tumors are associated with elevated 17-ketosteroids, but 17-ketosteroids produced by such tumors are independent of ACTH, and thus the urinary 17-ketosteroids are not markedly influenced by hydrocortisone steroids. When progestin therapy has been given prenatally as in cases of habitual abortion, and the child is born with signs of virilization, the 17-ketosteroids are normal and progressive virilization does not occur.

A prerequisite for hormone studies is determination of the base line urinary excretion of 17-ketosteroids, followed by administration of 10-25 mg. of fluorohydrocortisone daily in divided doses or equivalent amounts of prednisone, hydrocortisone, or cortisone for 4-5 days. Marked suppressibility of 17-ketosteroids excretion after such treatment means (usually) adrenal hyperplasia.[49, 50]

In 50 to 60% of the cases of Cushing's syndrome, adrenal hyperplasia is the underlying cause.[50] This may be the result of an excessive ACTH secretion by the Pituitary gland, or because of a pituitary tumor (more rare) or as a result of some primary dysfunction of the adrenal cortex. Thirty to forty percent of these cases are believed to be due to adenoma of the adrenal cortex with atrophy of the surrounding and contralateral gland. The remainder of cases, the least percentage are due to adrenocortical carcinoma. In this group there is a marked increase in the urinary excretion of 17-ketosteroids. The administration of cortisone diminishes the excretion of urinary 17-ketosteroids only in hyperplasia and has no influence in cases of adenoma and carcinoma.

In the past, reports has encouraged the determination of whether the elevated excretion of 17-ketosteroid is of alpha or beta configuration, but a recent study questions this procedure.[51]

REFERENCES

1. Higgins, C. C.: Urology—from 1905 to 1955. *Surg. Gynec. and Obst., 101:* 1-40, 1955.
2. Geshickter, C.: Suprarenal tumors. A. *J. Cancer, 23:* 104, 1935.
3. Goldzier, M. A.: *The Adrenals.* MacMillan Co., New York, 1929.
4. Langeron, L., and Lobeac, P.: Formes cliniques des tumeurs malignes primitive des capsules surrenales. *Ann. Med., 24:* 249, 1938.
5. Mathias, E.: Das Krankheitsbild des Interrenal's mus. *Med. Klin., 49:* 1879, 1929.
6. Meixner, K.: Zur Frage des Hermaphroditismus. *Zeitschr. Heilkunde, 26:* 318, 1905.
7. Loeb, M. J.: Adrenal cortical tumors. *Surg. Gynec. and Obst., 74:* 281, 1942.
8. Cahill, G. F., Melicow, M. M., and Darby, H. H.: Adrenal cortical tumors. *Surg. Gynec. and Obst., 74:* 281, 1942.
9. Soffer, L. J.: *Diseases of the Endocrine Glands.* Lea and Febiger, Philadelphia, 1958.
10. Williams, R. H.: *Textbook of Endocrinology.* Phila., W. B. Saunders Co., 1955.
11. Wilkins, L.: *Diagnosis and Treatment of Endocrine Diseases in Childhood and Adolescence.* Ed. 2, Thomas, Springfield, 1957.
12. Wilkins, L.: Masculinization of female fetus due to use of orally given progestins. *J.A.M.A.*, p. 118/1025, March 5, 1960.
13. Fordyce, A. D., and Evans, W. H.: Suprarenal virilism. *Quant. J. Med., 22:* 557, 1929.
14. Lisser, H.: Successful removal of adrenal cortical tumor causing sexual precocity in boy five years old. *Trans. Assoc. Amer. Phys., 48:* 224, 1933.
15. Cahill, G. F.: Adrenogenital syndrome and adrenal cortical tumors. *New England J. Med., 218:* 803, 1938.
16. Wilkins, L.: A feminizing adrenal tumor causing gynecomastia in a boy of five years contrasted with a virilizing tumor in a five-year-old girl. *J. Clin. Endocrinol., 8:* III, Feb. 1948.
17. Jolly, H. R.: Thesis. University of Cambridge, 1951.

18. Stone, R. K.: Extraordinary precocity in the development of the male sexual organs and muscular system of a child 4 weeks old. *A.M.J. Med. Sc., 24:* 561, 1952. Quoted by Jolly, H.: *Sexual Precocity.* Thomas, Springfield, 1955.
19. Reuben, M. S., and Manning, G. R.: *Arch. Pediat., 40:* 27, 1923. Quoted by Jolly, H.: *Sexual Precocity.* Thomas, Springfield, 1955.
20. Orel, H.: *Konst Lehre, 13:* 694, 1927-8. Quoted by Rush, H. P., Bilderback, J. B. Slocum, D., and Rogers, A.: *Endocrinology, 21:* 404, 1937.
21. Rush, H. P., Bilderback, J. B. Slocum, D., and Rogers, A.: *Endocrinology, 21:* 404, 1937. Quoted by Jolly, H.: *Sexual Precocity,* Thomas, Springfield, 1955.
22. Signst, E.: Vberdrei Falle von geniuner und einen Fall von zerebalar Pubertas praecox. *Paediat., 155:* 84, 1940.
23. Jacobsen, A. W., and Macklin, M. T.: Hereditary sexual precocity: report of a family with 27 affected members. *Pediatrics, 9:* 682, 1952.
24. Walker, S. H.: Constitutional true sexual precocity. *J. Pediat. 41:* 251, 1952.
25. Mortimer, H.: Quoted by Jolly, H.: *Sexual Precocity.* Thomas, Springfield, 1955.
26. Silagy, J. M., and Chiang, C. H.: Recent advances in the diagnosis and treatment of hermaphroditism and intersexuality. *New York State J. M., 58:* 280, 1958.
27. Jolly, H.: *Sexual Precocity.* Thomas, Springfield, 1959. American Lecture Series in Endocrinology No. 200.
28. Bing, J. F., Globus, J. H., and Simon, H.: *J. Mt. Sinai Hosp., 4:* 935, 1938. Quoted by Jolly, H.: *Sexual Precocity,* Thomas, Springfield, 1959. American Lecture Series in Endocrinology No. 200.
29. Weinberger, L. M., and Grant, F. C.: *Arch Int. Med., 67:* 762, 1941. Quoted by Jolly, H.: *Sexual Precocity.* Thomas, Springfield, 1959. American Lecture Series in Endocrinology No. 200.
30. Wilkins, L., Fleischmann, W., and Howard, J. E.: Macrogenitosomia precox associated with hyperplasia of the androgenic tissue of the adrenal and death from cortico-adrenal insufficiency. *Endocrinology, 26:* 358, 1940.
31. Patterson, J.: Diagnosis of adrenal tumors. *Lancet, 2:* 580, 1947.
32. Reeves, R. L., Tesluk, H., and Harrison, C. E.: Precocious puberty associated with hepatoma. *J. Clin. Endocrinol., 19:* 1651, 1959.
33. MacNab, G. H., Moncrieff, S. A., and Bodian, M.: Primary malignant hepatic tumors in childhood. In British Empire Cancer Campaign 3th Annual Report. Eastbourne, Sussex: Sumfield and Day Ltd., p. 168, 1952.
34. Case 46451; Weekly Clinico Pathological Exercises. Case Records of the Mass. Gen. Hosp. Editor, Castleman, B., *New England J. Med., 263:* 965, 1960.

35. Higgins, F., Brownlee, W. E., and Mantz, F. E., Jr.: Feminizing tumors of the adrenal cortex. *Amer. Surgeon, 22:* 56-79, 1956.
36. Wallach, S., Brown, H., Englert, E., Eik-Nes, K.: Adrenocortical Carcinoma with gynecomastia: Case Report and Review of Literature. *J. Clin. Endocrinol., 17:* 945-958, 1957.
37. Hinman, F., Steinbach, H. H., and Forsham, P. H.: Preoperative differentiation between hyperplasia and tumor in Cushing's syndrome. *J. Urol., 77:* 3, March, 1957.
38. Laragh, J. H.: The role of aldosterone in man. *J.A.M.A.*, Vol. 174, No. 3, Sept. 17, 1960, p. 293.
39. Deming, Q. B., and Luetscher, J. A., Jr.: Bioassay of desoxycorticosterone-like material in urine. *Proc. Soc. Exper. Biol. and Med., 73:* 171-175, Feb., 1950.
40. Simpson, S. A., et al.: Die Konstitution des Aldosterons: Uber Bestandteile der Nebennierenrinde und Verwandte Stoffe, Helvet. *Chim. Acta, 37:* 1200-1223, April, 1954.
41. Ulick, S., Laragh, J. H., and Lieberman, S.: Isolation of urinary metabolite of aldosterone and its use to measure rate of secretion of aldosterone cortex of man. *Tr. A. Am. Physicians, 71:* 225-235, 1958.
42. Editorial: Aldosterone secretion and blood pressure regulation. *J.A. M.A.*, Vol. 174, No. 3, p. 296, Sept. 17, 1960.
43. Hilton, J. G., Westerman, C. D., Bergen, S. S., and Crampton, R. S.: Syndrome of mineralo-corticoid excess due to bilateral adreno-cortical hyperplasia: Report of case. *New England J. Med., 260:* 202-205, Jan. 29, 1959.
44. Delmore, P., and Genest, J.: Primary aldosterone: Review of Medical literature from 1955 to June, 1958. *Canad. M.A.J., 81:* 893-902, Dec. 1, 1959.
45. Conn, J. W.: Primary aldosteronism, new clinical syndrome. *J. Lab. and Clin. Med., 45:* 3017, Jan., 1955.
46. Burke, A., and Liddle, G. W.: Virilizing adrenal hyperplasia. *South. M.J., 52:* 283-287, March, 1959.
47. Astwood, E. B., editor. *Progress in Clinical Endocrinology.* Grune and Stratton, Inc., New York, 1959.
48. Fisher, A. H., and Riley, C. L.: Preganediol excretion in a masculinizing syndrome. *J. Clin. Endocrin. and Med., 12:* 891, 1952.
49. Hallin, R. P., and Vix, V. A.: Virilism due to adrenal adenoma: Discussion of differential diagnosis. *Minnesota Med., 41:* 715-718, October, 1958.
50. Kuhl, W. J., and Lipton, M. A.: The diagnosis of adrenocortical disorders by laboratory methods. *New England J. Med.* Vol. 263, No. 3, p. 128-137, July 1960.
51. Gallagher, T. F.: Adrenocortical carcinoma in man: effect of amphenome on individual steroids. *J. Clin. Endocrinol., 18:* 937-949, 1958.

Chapter 12

TESTICULAR TUMORS

FEW SUBJECTS have been in such a permanent state of unrest as that of testicular tumors.[1] The association of testicular tumors and steroid hormones has engaged research workers in an ever-failing search for some clinical correlation. Recently, endocrinological studies, which formerly only seemed to have a vague research value, now seem to have great clinical significance. Unfortunately, most of the research experiments have been confined to laboratory animals, since it is not yet possible to apply many of the hypothetical theories to humans.

The testicles are synthetic stations for the manufacture of certain hormones. This mechanism is under the influence of the anterior lobe of the pituitary and hypophysis. Huggins[2] refers to the gonads (as well as the adrenal cortex and thyroid) as a "feed-back" mechanism which can inhibit the hypophyseal or pituitary influence, and that failure of "feed-back" mechanisms to operate, is one of the causes of hormonally induced cancer.

Chemical "feedback" is a relatively new concept. It is akin or likened to electronic "feedback," in that the end products of a series of chemical reactions are able to regulate their own production through "feedback" of a controlling signal.

Like other organs the testes are subject to tumor growths. As a rule such growths present the usual symptoms of neoplasia. Hormonal symptoms may or may not be present. In some instances, testicular tumors have definite alteration upon the hormonal status of the afflicted individual. This varies with age of onset of the disease and site of origin. For example a tumor of the interstitial cells of Leydig occurring in childhood manifests clinical symptoms of adolescent precocity and virilism, as evidenced by enlargement of the penis, male hiruitism, deeping of voice, and acceleration of muscular and skeletal development.[3,4,5] Paradoxically, the same type of tumor will produce in the adult male feminization with gynecomastia, loss of libido, and female hair and skin characteristics.

Why such an opposite hormonal function should occur has never been clearly explained. In the child, the precocious sexual behavior in the presence of such tumors has been attributed to an excessive production of androgen by the interstitial cells of Leydig. The opposite behavior of the same cell type of tumor in adults has led to the following explanations: (1) the tumors elaborate female hormones, (2) the tumors come from the Sertoli cells, the supposed origin of the testicular estrogens, (3) the tumors transfer androgens into estrogens, (4) estrogens are the cause, and not the result of the tumors, (5) the tumors decrease the normal androgen production, resulting in a predominance of estrogens, (6) the tumors elaborate abnormal hormones. No confirmation of these suppositions has been made as yet.[6, 7]

Sohval[8] believes that as a rule the etiologic mechanisms involved in the production of associated endocrinologic disturbances are not clear, but that in some cases, it is possible, that "testicular tumors may be the result rather than the cause of a hormonal dysfunction." This appears logical in view of the reported high incidence of testicular tumors in cryptorchidism and in male pseudohermaphrodites.

More recently Sohval[9] has applied this concept as an important factor in testicular neoplasia, based on the assumption, that there is reason to suspect that constitutional inferiority rather than abnormality of position may predispose a testicle to tumor formation. To quote Sohval, "There is reason to believe that an inherent defect of the testis itself, rather than its ectopic location, may predispose the undescended testicle to neoplasia. The present studies suggest that tubular immaturity in an adult's testicle, regardless of its location, may represent an anatomical expression of such a defect. It would thus appear that the same congenital imperfection which favors maldescent may also increase the likelihood of tumor development, similiar considerations may explain the occurrence of tumors in testes after they have been placed surgically in the scrotum."

At this point for sake of emphasis (see section on cryptorchism), the reader must be aware that orchiopexy or even spontaneous descent of the testis (hormonal treatment) has no lessening influence on the development of tumors in the cryptorchid. Testicular tumors have been reported in testes that have reached the scrotum by means of surgical intervention, as early as shortly after puberty, and in some as late as the fourth or fifth decade.

Barr's[10] identification and classification of nuclear sex chromatin study of the sex of testicular tumors has yielded some interesting results.[11, 12] Barr[13] himself has warned of the many problems associated with the interpretation of the nuclei of malignant cells. He has clearly pointed out that some of these difficulties are at present partly technical and partly because of their abnormal structure. He has advised to proceed cautiously with the interpretation of the nuclear sex of malignant tumors.

In 1954, Hunter[15] and Lennox sexed 8 testicular tumors and found 4 to be chromatin positive. These authors worked on the following assumptions: (1) If teratomata are simply ordinary tumors with unusually great capacities for differentiation in many directions, they should consist of tissues of the same sex as the host; (2) if, on the other hand, they are in any sense derived from separate individuals, the sex should sometimes be independent of that of the host. There was some doubt in the evaluation until a ninth case, of a pineal tumor, in a young male, a well differentiated "dermoid" was examined and found to have unmistakenly female nuclei. In this case subsequent examination of a skin biopsy raised considerable doubt about the nuclear sex of the patient. Myers[16] in discussing the nuclear sex of teratomas states that on rare occasions, a teratoma might develop in an apparently normal male, whose tissues contain female sex chromatin, for example, in Klinefelter's syndrome and related conditions. But this does not explain the relative frequent occurrence of female sex chromatin in testicular teratomas. Hunter[15] and Lennox have advanced a theory involving self-fertilization of two haploid cells (gametes or others) whereas others suggest the parthenogenetic divisions of haploid cells followed by chromosome duplication. Still others accept neither theory. Lennox[17] again has stressed the suggestion of the fusion of 2 haploid cells, claiming that it has an advantage in that it affords a possible explanation of the energy growth of the teratomata. "The fusion of the 2 haploids does seem to be a stimulus to subsequent growth, whereas there is no reason at all why the mere parthenogenetic divisions of a cell should cause active growth. There are arguments the other way, but I think there is still something in our original idea."

For the present it can only be said that the nuclear sex of tumors appears to be similar to the genetic sex.* Still unsolved remain many nuclear problems such as: teratomas in females are invariably female in nuclei; in males, only half are male, the remainder being chromatin positive. Clarification of this finding by chromosome studies will undoubtedly help to answer the question of the origin of these tumors.

General Discussion of Testis Tumors: Many classification of the testicular tumors have been offered. Many are misleading and confusing. As long ago as 1906, Chevassu[19] differentiated a relatively malignant growth, the seminoma, which he believed arose from the spermoblasts. Ewing refuted this, claiming that the unicellular seminoma is merely a one-sided development of a heterogenous growth to the exclusion of the other element. Ewing considered all tumors of the testicle to be teratoid.

Lewis[20] believes that a classification of testis tumors according to their morphological pattern as undifferentiated carcinoma, adenocarcinoma, papillary carcinoma and teratocarcinoma may

---

*That a chromatin mass is seen in tumor cells from female patients but is lacking in tumor cells from male patients has been repeatedly confirmed. In general, tumors have the chromosomal sex of their host. The following histogenic interpretation based on a study of 316 tumors is reported by Theiss, Ashley and Mostofi:[18] There are (3) modes of origin of gonadal tumors. (1) The stromal and interstitial cell tumors arise from diploid, non-germinal cells; (2) seminomas and dysgerminomas from germ cells before reduction division; and (3) teratomas and embryonal carcinomas from haploid germ cells by means of autofertilization. Of 25 ovarian teratomas, and 20 dysgerminomas, the nuclear sex was chromatin-positive, or of the same chromosomal sex of the host. Of 50 testicular seminomas, 25 interstitial cells, and 23 gonadal stromal cells, the nuclear sex was chromatin-negative and did not contain a sex chromatin mass. Some discrepancy was noted, such as in the teratomas and the embryonal carcinomas of the testis, a number reveal chromatin masses, were chromatin-positive, and thus not of the same chromosomal sex of the host.

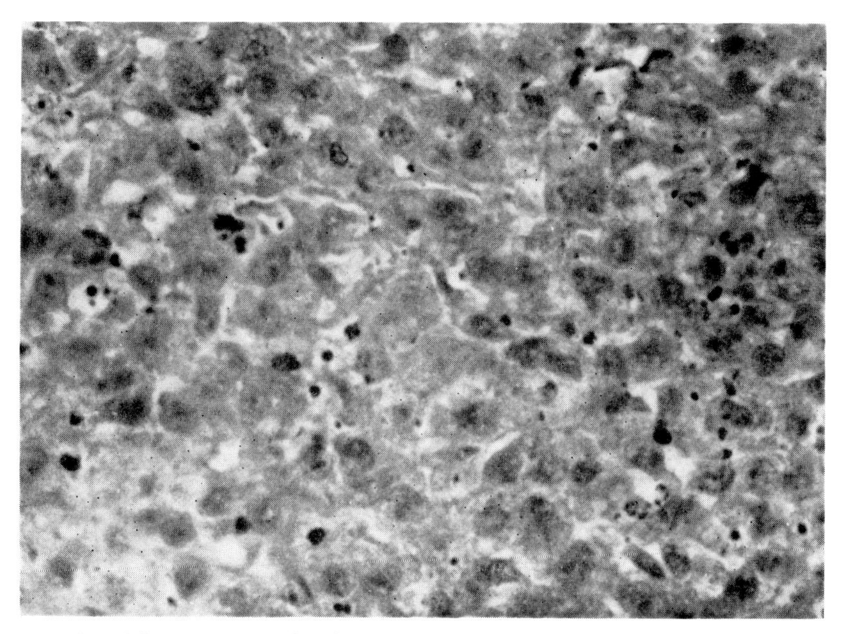

FIG. 31. Photomicrograph of a typical seminoma in testicle of a 50 year old white man who underwent orchiectomy because of painless swelling which had been present for at least 12 months. Note cells resembling lymphocytes, which are the most common type of secondary cellular elements in seminomas.

help the pathologist sort out his specimens but gives little aid to the clinician as to choice of a plan of therapy or opinion as to prognosis. "A division of this group of tumors into embryonal carcinoma and teratocarcinoma results in some benefit to the surgeon but there is no generally accepted concept as to what the terms imply."[20] A classification of testicular tumors as presented by Friedman[21] and Moore, has been adopted by the Army Institute of Pathology. The reader is referred to this classification as well as to the classification modified by Lewis,[20] and an additional modification by Melicow.[22]

Testicular tumors comprise 4% of all genito-urinary tumors. About 80% of these tumors occur in males under 40 years of age. In general it can be said that testicular tumors can be classified as to origin in growth, i.e., germinal which include seminoma,

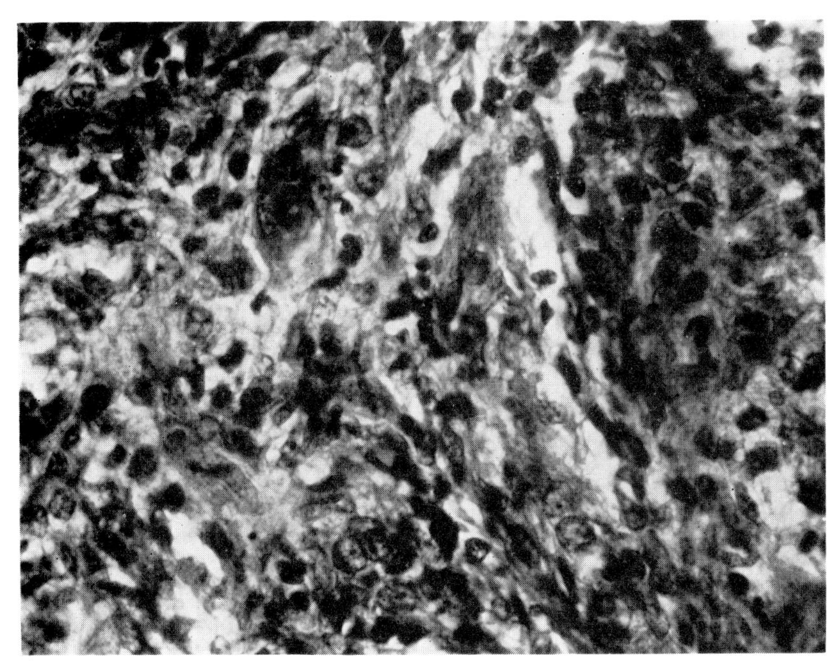

FIG. 32. Photomicrograph of Schistosomiasis of testicle of a 34 year old Puerto Rican man who underwent orchiectomy because of painless swelling which had been present for at least 3 months. Note tissue reaction to ova at 6 o'clock.

embryonic carcinoma, choriocarcinoma and terato-carcinoma; and non-germinal as capsular fibromas, interstitial cell tumors, androblastomas, adrenal cortical rests, adenomatoid tumors, tubular adnemomas and benign connective tissue tumors. The germinal cell tumor is the most prevalent (96%) and the non-germinal the least prevalent (4%). The germinal tumor originates from a toti-potent cell capable of differentiating in several trophoblastic directions. Moore[21] believes that the seminoma must be considered a germinal cell tumor because of its origin from intratubular tissue and resemblance to spermatogonia. Embryonic carcinomas demonstrate very early stages of differentiation of the toti-potent cells. Chorio-carcinomas are derived from the trophoblasts and cytotrophoblasts, whereas teratoma represents a more advanced differentiation with structures resembling fetal and adult tissues.

Seminomas are radio sensitive, whereas the remaining toti-potent tumors are radioresistant. Seminoma may be the precursor of embryonal carcinoma, teratocarcinoma and chorioepithelioma and may metastasize in such forms. Tumors of the testes metastasize first by lymphatics, but may metastasize by the blood stream. When early and lymphatic the metastases are unilateral and located in the lumbar nodes between the bifurcation of the common iliac arteries and the renal pedicle.

As stated earlier in this chapter, interstitial cell tumors in the adult are usually free of endocrine features. This is in contrast to its occurrence in infants and children when masculinization is the most striking symptom which usually calls attention to the tumor mass. Of course when a tumor mass is not palpable, macrogenito-

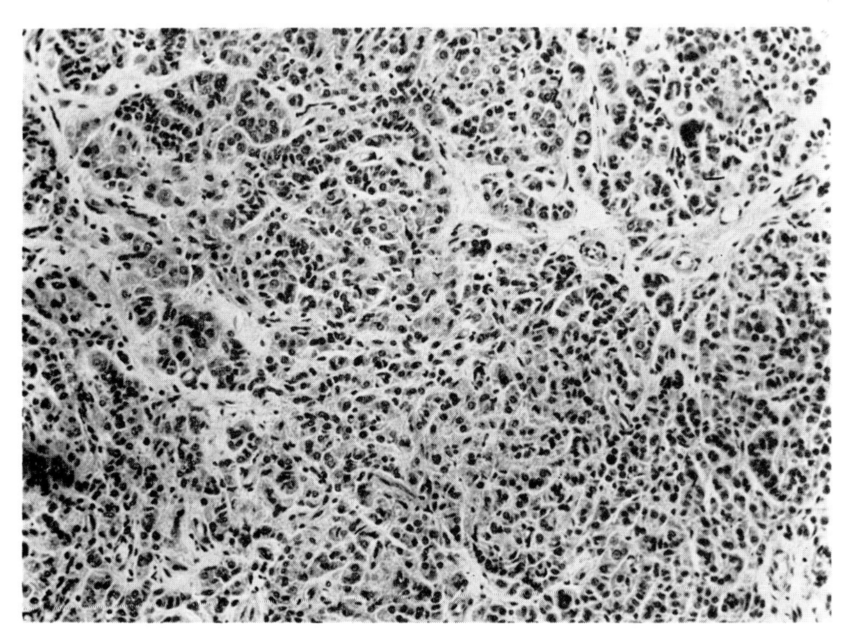

FIG. 33. Photomicrograph of testicle of 42 year old white male with typical local signs of testicular tumor with no clinical evidences of hormonal disturbances (gynecomastia is usually encountered in this type of tumor). Microscopically this lesion represents an interstitial cell tumor with areas of poor differentiation. The tumor is classified by some as "androblastoma," and by others as "gynandroblastoma" and by others as "interstitial cell tumor."

somia praecox caused by the interstitial cell tumor of the testes must be differentiated from congenital adrenal hyperplasia and adrenal cortical tumor. As stated in discussion of sexual precocity one always *suspects an adrenal cortical tumor in a male child if sexual precocity develops.* If testicular tumor mass can be ruled out, it is then necessary to distinguish between congenital adrenal hyperplasia and adrenal cortical tumor.

Of specific endocrinological significance is the unexplained hormonal findings in men with testicular tumors. Thus it has been shown that 75% of patients with testicular seminomas excrete increased amounts of follicle stimulating hormone (FSH) in the urine. Biologically this hormone is identical with that found in the urine of castrated or post-menopausal women. Of interest is that even after removal of the seminoma, the excretion of F.S.H. does not decrease and that there is no relation to the presence or absence of metastases. What is even more striking is that it has never been possible to demonstrate this hormone either in the tumor or in its metastases. For this reason it is inferred that the hormone in these cases is of pituitary origin.

The chorionic gonadotropin is not found in the urine of patients with seminoma but is found in the urine of men with teratomatous tumors. It is however only demonstrable in the presence of an active tumor, and disappears after the tumor is removed. Its appearance in the urine has been accepted as signifying the development of metastases, and generally indicates a poor prognosis.*

Estrogenic substances in the urine are occasionally elevated in testicular tumors, and is usually associated with increased excre-

---

*The explanation of hormone secretion in cases of testicular tumor is still varied and not universally standardized. Two types of gonadotropin are found in the urine of patients with certain testicular tumors. Thus one may find "chorionic" gonadotropin (identical biologic behavior as gonadotropin found in pregnancy urine) or a FSH gonadotropin. The chorionic gonadotropin has never been found in the urine of normal males, and only when a testicular tumor is present. The finding of high excretion levels of pituitary "castrate-like" gonadotropins (as in seminoma) has never been adequately explained, and it could easily be attributed to the tumor per se or the effect of the tumor. It cannot be likened to the effects of castration, since testicular tumors are usually unilateral. The belief that urinary gonadotropins decrease with successful surgery and reappear when metastases occurs, is not the rule in all cases, for metastases may be present without an increase in gonadotropin excretion, or the gonadotropin secretion may be high and the disease clinically cured.

tion of chorionic gonadotropins. Decrease in urinary androgens is found in patients with seminoma of the testis, but are not decreased as often or as markedly in cases of teratoma. The presence of "chorionic gonadotropic hormone" in the urine of a male is an indication of chorionic tumor tissue. Its increase may mean spread of the disease and its decrease may mean removal or regression of the tumor tissue.

Ever since Zondek[23] in 1928, reported finding gonadotropins in the urine of a patient with a testicular tumor, there has been no unanimity about the use and value of the test. When first announced there was great enthusiasm for the test, since it was erroneously assumed that all tumors of the testes would give a positive reaction. Melicow[22] and others feel that this test is an important procedure and should be utilized before operation in all cases and after operation when pathological findings prompt further testing. In Melicow's series of patients with testicular tumors, several developed gynecomastia. All gave negative Ascheim-Zondek reactions of the urine before surgery. It has been suggested that the positive Ascheim-Zondek test may be the result of an excess of gonadotropins elaborated by overactivity of the pituitary gland, uninhibited because of destruction of the remaining testes by tumor.

It has been universally believed that there was a direct relationship between atrophy of seminiferous tubules and hyperplasia of interstitial cells but this concept has been challenged. The findings of various independent studies tend to show that the number of Leydig cells changes are not the result of tubular atrophy. This then leaves the hormonal hypothesis as a possible explanation of hyperplasia and tumor formation, and that this could be the result of stimulation by the hypophysis or by biologically active neoplastic tissue. In this respect Twombly[24] and Pack have stated that tumors which elaborate large quantities of chorionic gonadotropius also seem to produce estrogens. It follows, that since both estrogenic substances and chorionic hormones can produce interstitial cell proliferation in experimental animals (and probably in man) it remains to identify one or the other of these substances as the underlying etiological agent. But most significant is that Leydig cell hyperplasia in association with testicular tumors is usually indicative of biologically active trophoblastic tissue.

The hazard of a second malignant tumor occurring in the remaining mate has been stressed by Harper *et al.*[25] These workers and others emphasize that when one testicle undergoes malignant changes there is a significantly greater hazard of a tumor developing in its mate. Indeed, it is recommended that any patient who has had a testicular cancer should have continued observations of the remaining gonad. Indeed this examination (periodic) should be carired on as long as the patient lives, for no one can deny that the remaining testis is a potential source of cancer.

The interstitial cells of Leydig play an important role in Interstitial Cell Tumors of the testicle. Though it is a rare tumor, the literature now seems to contain more of these cases than in former years. This may be due to improved clinical acumen rather than increase in the incidence of the tumor. As stated above tumors of the interstitial cells of Leydig are of two types: (1) tumors of the interstitial cells, which produce a virilizing effect (usually in male children); and (2) tumors of Leydig cells producing female sex hormones and feminization (usually in male adults).

The interstitial cells of Leydig arise from the stroma between the seminiferous tubules. These cells are believed to be the primary source of the male sex hormone. Hyperplasia of these cells is not uncommon and when it does occur it is usually associated with tubular atrophy. Simple hyperplasia occurs in chronic diseases, after vasectomy,* x-ray radiation, in cryptorchidism and in

*Experimental evidence tends to confirm the belief that vasecomy does not destory completely the gametogenic function of the testis. Histologic examination of testis subjected to vasoligation reveal that many of the seminiferous tubules contain gametogenic cells. Some of the tubules do degenerate and it is assumed that the tubules alternately degenerate and repair.

As early as 1903 it was reported that vasoligation would destroy the spermatogenic tissue of the testis and lead to hypertrophy of the interstitial cells of Leydig. This gave rise to the hypothesis of rejuvenation in 1920 in which it was contended that: 1) vasoligation of domestic animals and man destroys the seminal epithelium but increases the cells of Leydig; 2) the increase in number and size of the interstitial cells of Leydig produces an increased amount of male sex hormone; and 3) this release of increased androgens would "rejuvenate" the depleted male.

The actual effect of vasectomy, other than sterilization, is still imperfectly understood.

local inflammatory conditions. A clear distinction between interstitial cell hyperplasia and interstitial cell tumor is not always practical or possible. The tumor is often referred to as androblastoma or Sertoli cell tumor. Mostofi[18] and his associates prefer to call these tumors, "specialized gonadal stromal tumor." Teilum[26, 27] designates these tumors as androblastomas, derived in either sex from undifferentiated gonadal mesenchyme and which histologically reflect the various phases in the development of the male gonad. Teilum groups interstitial cell tumors of the testis and luteomas, masculinoblastomas and "adrenal tumors" of the ovary, under one heading, namely, "virilizing diffuse androblastomas."

The excellent account of the histopathology of these tumors by Dixon[28] and Moore is strongly recommended to the interested reader. The tumor is considered benign, but as emphasized by Dixon and Moore, the possibility exists of malignant variants of androblastoma, as indicated by the not infrequent occurrence of malignant arrhenoblastomas.*

When present in a child they are characterized by precocious sexual development and must be differentiated from other causes of precocious puberty. Thus they assume great importance to the urologist who must recognize and identify the specific cause of the disorder.

These children exhibit the following endocrine changes: Change in voice, distribution of body hair similar to adult distribution, muscular development similar to adult development, mental maturity, adult sexual activities including erections and ejaculations and spermatozoa in the ejaculate. In approximately 15% of the recorded cases of adults, gynecomastia and loss of libido were reported.

Most instructive is the report of Rezek[4] and Hardin of a case of bilateral interstitial cell tumor observed over a period of 14 years:

---

*Most of the reported cases have been histologically and clinically benign. Microscopically they are made up of uniform, large, polyhedral, liver-like cells with abundant eosinophilic granular cytoplasm containing brown pigment, sudanophilic vacuoles and at times Reinke's crystalloids, which may at times also be found in normal interstitial cells. As a rule these tumors are definitely demarcated but are not encapsulated.

At age 6 this patient had the stature and facial characteristics of an adolescent male. The genitalia were the size of an adult's. Three years later the left testicle was 10 times normal size, felt heavy and did not transilluminate. At this time the right testis was also enlarged but not as enlarged as the left one. X-ray studies revealed a bone age of 18. The sella turcica was not abnormal. Following orchiectomy (left) regression of precocious development occurred. Eight years later when the patient was seventeen, he was described as being stocky and well developed. At this time the right testis was 3 x normal size and hard and nodular, and biopsy revealed a benign interstitial cell tumor. A right orchiectomy was performed when the patient was 19 years of age and findings confirmed findings of testicular tumor, namely benign interstitial cell tumor. The author's report the patient at 20 to be living a normal life on testosterone therapy, with hair distribution, voice and muscular development within normal range. These authors stress the significance of variations in 17-ketosteroid determinations reported in the literature. "However, in our case," they state, "we show an interesting curve in the 17-ketosteroid determinations. The initial test was taken after the first orchiectomy and was about nine times the normal, with the beta portion being greater than the alpha. Then it was observed that following the removal of the second testicle the values dropped to normal or subnormal with the beta portion disappearing completely. The disappearance of the beta portion may be explained on the basis that the source (the testicles) were removed. Also there must be a factor in the testicle that stimulates the adrenals causing an elevation of the alpha portion, because after removal of the testicles, the portion again becomes normal. Whether this is a typical curve remains to be seen."

Variations in the 17-ketosteroids determinations reported in the literature are as follows: Masson and Venning,[29] Reiners and Horne[30] reported normal values before surgery. Newns,[31] Reiners[29] and Sandbloom[31] observed elevation before surgery and return to normal after surgery (orchiectomy).* When the Fried-

*Despite these accounts, interstitial cell tumors have been reported to produce enormous amounts of androgens. Excess production of androgens in teratomas is probably the result of interstitial cell secretion. In other testicular tumors it would be more logical to assume that there would be little change from the normal.

man tests were performed they were reported as negative by Garvey, Melicow, Reiners, Stewart and Grabstald.[32] These inconsistent findings do not help to clarify the clinical picture of interstitial cell tumor of the testis with regard to 17-ketosteroid excretion and hormone excretion.

A singular contribution to a better understanding of interstitial cell tumor of the testes is that of Delgard[33] and Hesselberg who report two cases and survey and report on 94 reported cases from the literature. These authors like many of the American authors emphasize the importance of distinguishing between interstitial cell hyperplasia and interstitial cell tumor. They state, "An increased number of interstitial cells between more or less preserved tubules (hyperplasia) is a rather common occurrence, i.e., in cryptorchid testicle, in atrophic testicular tissue compressed by a hydrocele, a tumor or an infectious granuloma, following orchitis, ligature of the deferent duct, trauma to the gonad or radiation etc. In these cases the primary lesion involves testicular atrophy. This, presumably, through decreased endocrine activity exerts a (secondary) stimulation of the anterior pituitary, with increased production of the interstitial cell stimulating hormone (ICSH) which in turn is followed by a (tertiary) interstitial cell hyperplasia. In true interstitial cell tumors on the contrary, a primary neoplastic process displaces the seminiferous tubules."

Tumors of the Sertoli Cells (Feminization): Tumors of the Sertoli cells are rare but of significant hormonal importance.[34, 35, 36] In the dog, this type of tumor is quite common and often will cause feminization.* Some authorities believe that many so-called tubular adenomas (a similarly rare testicular tumor) were probably Sertoli cell tumors.[37] Sovahl[8] describes only 1 case reported in a normal male by Teilum.[38] The phenomenon of feminization is believed to be due to marked estrogenic excretion by the Sertoli cells. Teilum[38] described the histological appearance of the tumor to be identical with that of ovarian arrhenoblastoma and though

*In 1952, Dixon and Moore reviewed the files of the Armed Forces Institute of Pathology thru 1947 and stated: "It is worthy of note that in our series we found no Sertoli cell tumors, indicating that there may be no human homologue of the Sertoli cell tumors seen so frequently in dogs."

morphologically alike the hormonal action is quite different. Thus the testicular tumor manifests itself by feminization of the afflicted male, whereas the ovarian arrhenoblastoma, manifests itself by masculinization of the afflicted female. The latter is believed to be due to androgen-producing precursors of Leydig cells, whereas in the former due to estrogen-producing Sertoli cells. Lewis[39] and Stockard have reported a feminizing tumor of the testis in which increased amounts of urinary pregnanediol and chorionic gonadotropin was found.

Treatment: "The management of tumors of the testis is by no means a settled issue. Surgery and x-ray have improved the outlook for many of these unfortunate individuals, but the results to date still leave much to be desired. Undoubtedly there is still room for improvement in surgical technique and application of irradiation."[40] The following policy is recommended:

(1) In cases of seminoma, orchiectomy is followed by irradiation therapy to the abdominal lymphatic chain.

(2) In cases of embryonal carcinoma and teratocarcinoma, in the absence of clinical metastasis, orchiectomy is followed by bilateral lymphadenectomy performed through a trans peritoneal approach. However if the nodes removed are negative pathologically no additional irradiation is given. Nevertheless if the node or nodes removed reveal metastasis, post operative irradiation is applied to the entire lymphatic chain, including the left supraclavicular region area, mediastinum and abdomen.

(3) Patients with choriocarcinoma are subjected to high orchiectomy only. Lymphadenectomy and/or irradiation is fruitless.

(4) Patients with adult teratomas are treated by orchiectomy and lymphadenectomy, followed by irradiation if the nodes are positive.

REFERENCES

1. Gonder, M. J., and Fadell, E. J.: Gonadal stromal tumor in an infant. *J. Urol.*, 84, p. 357-359, 1960.
2. Huggins, C.: Endocrine factors in Cancer. *J. Urol., 68:* 875-885, 1952.
3. Di George, A. M., and Paschkis, K. E.: Tumors of the testis. *Pediat. Clinics of North Amer., 6:* 604, 1959.

4. Rezek, P., and Hardin, H. C., Jr.: Bilateral interstitial cell tumor of the testicle. Report of a case observed 14 years. *J. Urol., 74:* 628, 1955.
5. Herbut, P. A.: Urologic Pathology. Philadelphia, Lea and Febiger, 1952.
6. Warren, S., and Olshausen, K. W.: Interstitial cell growths of the testicle. *Am. J. Path., 19:* 307, 1943.
7. Eisendadt, H. B., and Petry, J. L.: Testicular interstitial cell tumor with feminization in the adult male. *J. Urol., 78:* 428-434, 1957.
8. Sohval, A. R.: Diseases of the Testis. Chapter 17, in Soffer, J. L.: *Diseases of the Endocrine Glands.* Lea and Febiger, Philadelphia, 2nd edition, 1958.
9. Sohval, A. R.: Testicular dysgenesis in relation to neoplasm of the testicle. *J. Urol., 75:* 2, 1956.
10. Barr, M. L.: The skin biopsy test of chromosomal sex in clinical practice. *Anat. Rec., 121:* 387, 1955.
11. Myers, L.: The nuclear sex of teratomas. *Symposium on Nuclear Sex.,* p. 142, Inter Science Publishers, Inc., New York, 1958.
12. Tavares, S. A.: Further inquiries into the sex of tumors. *Symposium On Nuclear Sex,* p. 160, Inter Science Publishers, Inc., New York, 1958.
13. Atkin, B. N.: Observations on sex chromatin in human tumors. *Symposium on Nuclear Sex,* p. 168, Inter Science Publishers, Inc., New York, 1958.
14. Barr, M. L.: Concluding remark. *Symposium on Nuclear Sex,* p. 181, Inter Science Publishers, Inc., New York, 1958.
15. Hunter, W. F., and Lennox, B.: Quoted by Tavares, S. A.: Further inquiries into the sex of tumors. *Symposium on Nuclear Sex,* p. 160, Inter Science Publishers, Inc., New York, 1958.
16. Myers, L. M.: The Nuclear Sex of Teratomas. *Symposium on Nuclear Sex,* p. 143, Inter Science Publishers, Inc., New York, 1958.
17. Lennox, B.: In comment on presentation, The Sex Chromatin, Lennox, B., Serr, D. M., and Ferguson-Smith, M. A., in Memoirs of the Society for Endocrinology, No. 7, Cambridge, 1960.
18. Mostofi, F. K., Theiss, E. A., and Ashley, D. J. B.: Tumors of specialized gonadal stroma in human male patients. *Cancer, 12:* 944-957, 1959.
19. Chevassau, M.: *Tumeurs du Testicule.* Paris, 1906. (Paris Thèses, 1905-1906).
20. Lewis, L. G.: Testis tumors: report on 250 cases. *J. Urol., 59:* 763, 1948.
21. Friedman, N. B., Moore, R. A.: Tumors of testis: report of 922 cases. *Military Surg., 99:* 573, 1946.
22. Melicow, M. M.: Classification of tumors of testis: A clinical and pathological study based on 105 primary and 13 secondary cases

in adults, and 3 primary and 4 secondary cases in children. *J. Urol., 73:* 547, 1955.

23. Zondek, B.: Gonadotropic hormone in diagnosis of chorioepithelioma. *J.A.M.A., 108:* 607, 1937.
24. Twombly, G. H., and Pack, G.: Relationship of Hormones to Testicular Tumors. In *Endocrinology of Neoplastic Diseases.* Oxford University Press, New York, 1947.
25. Harper, H., Quoted by Myers, L. M. in The Nuclear Sex of Teratomas. Symposium on Nuclear Sex. Inter Science Publishers, New York, 1958.
26. Teilum, G. Estrogen-producing Sertoli cell tumors (androblastoma tubulare lipoides) of human testis and ovary; homologous ovarian and testicular tumors. III. *J. Clin. Endocrinol., 9:* 301-318, 1949.
27. Teilum, G.: Classification of testicular and ovarian androblastoma and Sertoli cell tumors. *Cancer, 11:* 769-782, 1958.
28. Dixon, F. S., and Moore, R. A.: Testicular tumors: Clinico pathological study. *Cancer,* 427-454, 1953.
29. Mason, P., and Venning, E. H.: Tumeur Maligni des cellules de Leydig. *Rev. Canad. de Biol., 1:* 571, 1942.
30. Reiners, Jr., Charles R., and Horn, Jr., Robert C.: Interstitial cell tumor of the testis. *Am. J. Clin. Path., 19:* 1039, 1949.
31. Newns, G. H.: Precocious sexual development due to an interstitial cell tumor of the testis. *Brit. J. Surg., 39:* 379, 1952. Reiners, C. R. Reference No. 30. Sandblom, P.: Precocious sexual development produced by an interstitial cell tumor of the testis. *Acta Endocrinol., 1:* 107, 1948.
32. Grabstald, H.: Testicular endocrinopathy in clinical urology. *J. Urol., 76:* 609-624, 1956.
33. Dalgard, J. B., and Hesselberg, F.: Interstitial cell tumors of the testis; two cases and survey. *Acta. Path. et Microbiol. Scandinav., 41:* 219, 1957.
34. Huggins, C., and Moulder, P. V.: Estrogen production by Sertoli cell tumors of the testis. *Cancer Research, 5:* 510, 1945.
35. Mulligan, R. M.: Feminization in male dogs. *Am. J. Path., 20:* 865, 1944.
36. Rewell, R. E.: Tubular adenoma of testis and asterogenic activity, *J. Path. and Bact., 59:* 321, 1947.
37. Stalker, A. L., and Hendry, W. T.: Hyperplasia and Neoplasia of the Sertoli cell. *J. Path. and Bact., 64:* 161, 1952.
38. Teilum, G.: Arrhenoblastoma-androblastoma, homologous ovarian and testicular tumors. *Acta. Path. et Microbiol. Scandin. 23:* 252, 1946.
39. Lewis, L. G., and Stockard, C. G.: Feminizing testis tumors. *J. Urol., 64:* 518, 1950.
40. Patton, S. F., and Mallis, N.: Tumors of the testis. *J. Urol., 81:* 457, 1959.

Chapter 13

TRANSVESTISM

MANY WILL question the inclusion of a subject such as transvestism in a text, basically devoted to the Biology of the Human Testes. But a biological treatise means a study of life in all its forms and phenomena, particularly with reference to origin, growth, development, structure and behavior. It is not my purpose to deal with problems of abnormal sexual behavior or sexual perversions since such abnormalities are entirely independent of a testicular anatomical abnormality. However, it cannot be denied that certain abnormal sexual patterns are the result of faulty sex assignment, particularly when the assignment is reversed on several occasions. The remarkable advances made within recent years in cytogenetics, embryology and biochemistry have changed many of the concepts of sexual anomalies in man and stimulated great doubt as to many of our present theories concerning sexual behavior. Faulty hormonal influence of sex differentiation may play a greater role in certain forms of abnormal sexual behavior than has heretofore been accepted. This is applicable to transvestism, in which the role of the gonads in an abnormal sexual behavior requires further clarification.

Transvestism is an old afflicition of mankind. It has been known in all cultures and in all parts of the world. Herodetes describes it as the mysterious "Skythian illness" found on the north shores of the Black Sea, where normal men would put on female clothes, do female work and act in every way of mannerism and behavior as a female. This strong desire and sense of longing to wear the garments of a female (it is not confined to the male and there are many female transvestites who wish to wear the garments of a male) was known in ancient Rome. Indeed it was quite prevalent at the time of Romes's decline when some of the Roman Emperors occasionally dressed in female garments.

Transvestism, also known as "eonism" undoubtedly received this particular name from the often narrated stories of the proverbial Chevalier d'Enode Beaumont. Beaumont was a diplomatic agent of Louis XV and was believed to be a woman but proved at post-mortem to be a man. Hirschfield[1] in his work, "The Transvestites," delightfully records the story of this remarkable person, who was the secret correspondent of Louis XV, and who lived to be 83 years of age, 49 as a man and 34 as a woman. The arguments as to his sex were carried on for decades and it has been reported that in England the wagers amounted to more than 200,000 pounds. In France 80,000 francs was wagered on the same issue.

Some authorities associated transvestism to homosexual tendencies. Krafft-Ebing[2] believed it to be a variant of homosexuality. It is a condition which occurs independently and must be considered separately from any other sexual anomaly. Hirschfield differed with Krafft-Ebing and his school. Stekel[3] attacked Hirschfield for his views and wrote: "Those who draw a distinction between transvestism and homosexuality do violence to the facts." In reply to which Hirschfield answered that "It may be that in transvestites, *as in everybody without exception*– (italics mine), the homosexual pattern hidden or repressed in the subconscious can ultimately be dragged to light by psychoanalysis. For clinical consideration however, latent impulses are not so important as manifest impulses, and there can be no doubt at all that to many transvestites homosexuality is subjectively just as repellent as to the majority of heterosexuals."

In this respect a more modern view is presented by Armstrong[4] who emphasizes that transvestism may be symptomatic of homosexuality and occasionally of other sexual perversions, but only a small minority of homosexuals are transvestites. "And transvestism as applied to cases such as described, i.e., eonism, is a phenomenon quite distinct from homosexuality. The two are frequently confused even by psychiatrists and psycho-analysts."

Armstrong (who kindly sent me the accompanying photograph) describes a most instructive case of transvestism, which has been fully investigated and presented at a Symposium on *Nuclear Sex*.[4] It is so typical that I am quoting it verbatum:

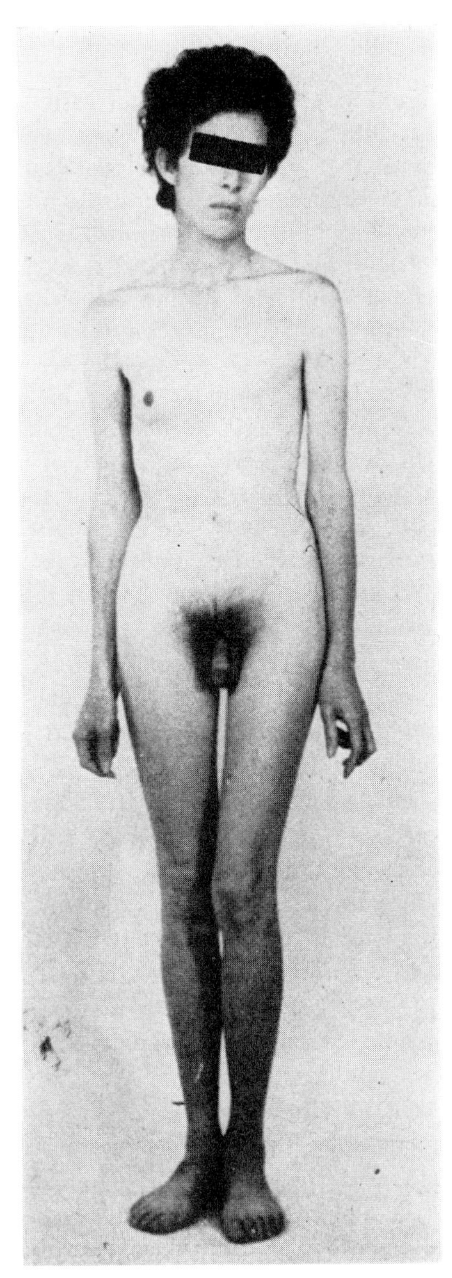

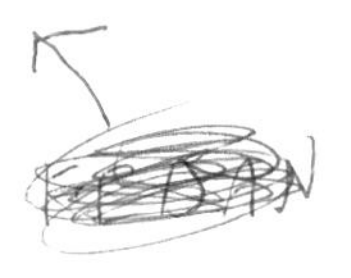

Fig. 34. Male transvestite.—Male aged 28 with slender and graceful physique, with smooth and almost hairless facial expressions characteristically feminine. Left breast removed for growth when patient was 21 years of age. Genitalia normal except for small testes. *(From Armstrong, C. N.:* Transvestism, *1958. Courtesy of Interscience Publishers, Inc.)*

Male, aged 28, occupation, cook. As a child was healthy and free from neurotic traits. He has a detailed memory for his early life and would appear from an early age to have a strong preference for girl's games and chose girls as his playmates. Already at the age of three or four he had begun to dress in feminine clothes on every possible occasion despite strong disapproval from his parents, brother and sister. He would go to school dressed as a boy and as soon as he arrived home would change into girl's clothes. On leaving school he worked for a year at a corset factory and then was apprenticed to a piano tuner with whom he worked for five years. At this time he adopted certain feminine features in his dress to which his mother made very strong objections, and he experienced cruelty and ridicule from society on account of his femininity. During the past four years he has worked as a waiter and chef.

He has always identified himself with girls and the feeling that he is a woman compelled by society to live and act as a man has dominated his life. His tense belief that he is essentially female issues partly from the fact that he is convinced that he has never had to make conscious efforts to imitate female gestures and mannerisms or efforts to imitate female gestures and mannerisms or affect an interest in feminine activities. These things have come to him with a spontaneity of instructive attributes. He expresses hatred of and revulsion from the outward signs of masculinity in his sexual organs and considers he has a right to have them removed so that he can approximate more closely to feminine anatomy, and can live as a woman without a feeling of deceit that is repugnant to him, or a fear of discovery and persecution. At present he is denied all possibility of friendship, whereas if he were not so indubitably male he would be able to achieve platonic relationships with either men or women.

He has never had desire for normal or perverse sexual intercourse but several times he has become romantically infatuated with virile men. His love for these men has been intense and deep, but of a purely platonic nature. The thought of sexual physical contact with men or women disgusts him, yet he has indulged in fantasies of pregnancy and has had a passionate desire for motherhood.

> On clinical examination the patient's physique was slender and graceful, his skin smooth and almost wholly hairless and his face mobile and expressive. His gestures and mannerisms, as well as his facial expressions, were feminine in what strikes one as a spontaneous and unaffected manner. His weeping, which was witnessed a number of times at interview, was feminine too in the high pitch of the cry, the abundance of tears, the prolonged loss of control and the change of expression."
>
> What was most significant was that on examination the penis and testicles were small. Although facial hair was present it was definitely deficient for a male of his age and the pubic hair, although reaching to the umbilicus was below standard. Gynecomastia was present on the right side. The left breast had been removed for a growth when the patient was 21 years of age. Oral mucosa smears from both cheeks were chromatin negative. Bilateral testicular biopsy revealed atrophic testicular tissue with complete absence of spermatogenesis, scanty interstitial cells, marked fibrosis and thickening of the basement membrane of the seminiferous tubules. The urinary 17-ketosteroids were 1.3 mg. in 24 hours.

Lukianowicz[5] has written an excellent modern survey of the various aspects of Transvestisim. This is a splendid article, and the interested reader is urged to consult with this paper. Lukianowicz uses the term "transvestism" for a sexual deviation characterized by; (a) a desire to wear the dress of the opposite sex and; (b) (less often) a wish to be looked upon, and to be socially accepted, as a member of this sex. "The name 'trans-sexualism' is applied to these rare cases of transvestism, where, apart from both just mentioned tendencies, there exists; (c) a persistent morbid urge to undergo a 'conversion-operation,' i.e., to have anatomical 'change' of the inborn sex."

The problem of transvestism is an extremely difficult one mainly because of the diversity of opinion concerning the etiological factors in this strange disorder. There seems to be two lines of thought, namely (a) that it is biologic or having a genetic and endocrine origin, (b) that it is the result of an early psychological experience.

(a) Genetic and endocrine theory: This theory seems to be most favored by the endocrinologists. It is based on the assump-

tion that the chromosomal, or "genetic" sex (found in the nuclear structure of all body cells) does not always correspond to the respective gonadal, or "endocrine" sex. Thus an "endocrine" male may be a genetic female and similarly an "endocrine" female may be a genetic male. All of which may result in an inverted psycho-sexual make-up. But the matter is not that simple for as a result of the work of Moore,[6, 7, 8, 9] Graham and Barr and others, male transvestites have typical male-type chromatin nuclei. In this respect these cases closely resemble cases of Klinefelter's[10, 11, 12, 13] syndrome in which individuals of a male phenotype have chromatin negative nuclei although the majority of cases of Klinefelter's syndrome reveal chromatin positive nuclei.

It is well to subject these cases to testicular biopsy whenever possible. In many cases the patients have been under estrogenic therapy. In the cases described by Armstrong,[4] the patient told him that he had never taken estrogens or other similiar medication, in fact would not know how to obtain same. Bilateral testicular biopsy of this patient revealed thickening of the basement membranes of the tubules, edema of the interstitial tissue and an apparent arrest of spermatogenesis at the spermatid stage. Such findings tend to confirm the belief that although the etiology of the condition is obscure, the specific factor is likely to be constitutional and on a genetic basis.

(b) Psychological: No one can deny that psychiological factors contribute in causation. Those who advocate the theory of psychological conditioning believe that an adverse psychological conditioning in childhood leads to the development of transvestism. Thus parental rejection of a child because of his undesired sex undoubtedly can lead to feelings of inferiority, insecurity and a confused conception of the problems of masculinity and femininity. Thus patients are prone to say, "had I been a boy everything would have been all right," or "had I been a girl, things would have been different." The literature abounds with cases, where the afflicted person having been rejected by their parents for their sex develop a hostile, sadomasochistic attitude towards their own genitalia. "They direct their resentment and their hatred to this visible 'cause' of their rejection and unhappiness, and want to have

them," (1), either hidden under the dress of the sex to which their parents wanted them to belong, and which they try by their cross-dressing to represent (transvestites); or (2), completely removed (and possibly supplanted by sexual organs of the opposite sex, by means of a 'conversion-operation' (trans-sexualists). In this way both types endeavor to acquire the acceptance and love of their rejecting parents."[14]

In this respect Lukianowicz[5] writes of his patient as saying, "I hated the fact that I had male organs." Warden and Marsh[15] state all their patients, "had a rejecting attitude toward their own genitalia, regarding them as objects of contempt and ugliness, several said they had masturbated to destroy the genitals." Indeed many make serious attempts at self-mutilation as demonstrated by the following case admitted to the Urologic service at the Flower-Fifth Avenue Hospital.

> L. B., a 30 year old white male night club worker, was admitted to the hospital thru the emergency room after intentionally cutting off part of his penis and testicles. Patient came to psychiatric clinic for advice concerning his confusion about sex and when unable to see a physician went to lavatory and with a sharp knife amputated part of his penis and part of scrotum including both testicles, which he discarded into toilet bowl. In emergency room patient presented a denuded proximal portion of penis approximately 2½ inches in external length, the distal end of which shows a clear, complete amputation with both corpora cavernosa and spongiosa with contained urethra in normal relationships.
>
> The antero-superior aspect of the scrotal sac was partially amputated. The skin edges were completely retracted, exposing the floor of both scrotal sacs. The cut margin of the scrotal sac was continuous with the cut margin of the skin suprapubically, at which point there was an area approximately one inch in width devoid of skin, completely encircling the dorsal surface of the penis. Scrotal contents (testes and attached cord) were not visible in the open wound and it appeared at this time, that there had been total emasculation. A revision of the penis and scrotum was subsequently performed and the patient was then transferred to Bellevue for psychiatric observation.

When the patient was first discovered, he was wearing silk stockings and a woman's slip and dress and claimed his name to be Louise. After shock treatment for hemorrhage was instituted and patient reached ward, he intelligently responded to questions. He stated that since childhood he has desired to be a woman. He first wore female clothes at 8 and 9 years of age. As he grew older he tried to forget this urge and even dated girls but always felt like a female. He enlisted (has tatooed arms) and was discharged from the Marines, when found dressed in female clothing. He was under observation in the Naval Hospital, also at the Boston Mental Health Center. He lives alone and when home always wore woman's clothes. He was desirous of having a sex adjustment operation, and felt he could no longer resist desire for emasculation and hence his obvious apparent success at so doing it himself. He admitted to heterosexual and homosexual relations and lack of enjoyment with both. He has difficulty in making friends and unable to concentrate at work because of great desire to wear female clothes. As a child he never felt secure. His parents were extremely strict. He has one sister, 36–married and one child–one sister, 28, considered to be neurotic, and one brother, 12, in good health. *Here then is a case of transvestism with a drastic attempt at destruction of the hated sexual organ.*

Lukianowicz[5] brings into his excellent discussion on Transvestism a third theory of explanation, namely: (c) The Psychoanalytical Theory. He states, "All psychoanalytically minded writers base their interpretations of transvestism on the teaching of Freud." "Their point of view," states Lukianowicz, "may be summarized thus: transvestism is an attempt to overcome the fear of castration by creating an imaginary phallic woman, and subsequent identification with her. This fear of castration and its denial through creation of a phallic woman is often precipitated by an exhibitionistic behavior of the important female figure in the transvestites early childhood, representing most often his mother or his sister." Bak[6] accepts and emphasizes the disturbance of the mother-child relationship, resulting in an alternating identification with the phallic and penisless mother, with the corresponding split in the ego. Of singular interest is that such explanation cannot be applied to female transvestites. Thus if transvestism is a symbolic denial of castration fear through creation of a phallic woman, how can one explain female transvestism?

Greene[17] describes a case of "acute transvestism" in which the patient during the day had a great desire of wanting to appear as a woman. During the night he dreamed fantasies of being a woman. He was tough, rugged individual, described as a hard drinking and happily married man. He rapidly developed gynecomastia and the above symptoms of transvestism. He was given three injections of testosterone propionate and the gynecomastia diminished but persisted sufficient to warrent further investigation. This revealed that he was suffering from cirrhosis of the liver and Greene concluded that the mental symptoms and gynecomastia were due to a failure of the liver to conjugate his circulating estrogens.

Several cases of Klinefleter's disease have been described with hetrosexual tendencies. Sieberman[18] speaks of one case of Klinefelter's syndrome with female trends and which paradoxically revealed evidence of spermatogenesis by testicular biopsy studies. Davidson[19] tells of the following interesting case:

"His mother was a most unsatisfactory person, a drunkard who disappeared from home for several months at a time. As a boy he had always been called sissy, and eventually when he left school he drifted through various employments and the only ones he held for any length of time was of an artistic nature. We examined his blood and found that he had drum-sticks in the leukocytes. He looked a female, assumed female attitudes and had even got a wide carrying angle, but he had well formed male external genitals apart from the small size of the testes. Further examination, including a testicular biopsy, confirmed that he was a case of true Klinefelter's syndrome." This patient was in a confused psychological state, had difficulty making the necessary adjustments to life and on several occasions tried to commit suicide. Davidson[19] believed this case to represent another variety of transvestism with the possibility that he might also be a true hermaphrodite.

Bishop[20] speaks of a similar case of transvetism who was also a Klinefelter with female genetic sex, and raises the legal point of sentencing such a person for having homosexual relations.

Bakwin[21] in a plea to pediatricians emphasizes that transvestism is more common in boys than in girls and that it is usually first noted in the fourth year, though probably begins earlier. He recommends that treatment should begin as early as possible to make the diagnosis, and that the first step to a detailed review of the home situation, with special attention to the parent's attitude to one another and to the child. The dominating mother should be curbed, and the too-passive father should be encouraged to take a more active part in the child's life. At all times the young patient should be encouraged in the behavior that is characteristic of his sex and discouraged from behaving like the opposite sex. Teasing and shaming are not recommended, are ineffective and may even be harmful by raising the child's negativism. Confusion about sex must be clarified and explanation given in a simple manner which the child can understand. All recommend psychiatric help and guidance, particularly if parental resistance is encountered or the child's behavior seems deeply intrenched and does not respond to general suggestions. Treatment for the adult transvestite is more difficult and less satisfactory. Most resent the implication that they may have homosexual tendencies. On the other hand, the young male transvestite may be driven to associate with male homosexual circles because of confusion or because they find understanding in such circles.[23]

Wilkins, states that transvestism is not due to hormonal abnormality. In fact he classifies this disorder as a homosexual orientation. "Transvestites," states Wilkins, "are almost without exception, physically and hormonally normal. They trace their transvestic interests back to pre-school years." In this respect it should also be noted that Wilkins believes that homosexual orientation probably depends in some way or the other upon rearing and the kind of sex experiences a person encounters and transacts but that this formula of encounters and transactions that produces homosexuality has not as yet been deciphered.[25]

SUMMARY

(1) Transvestism is a condition too often erroneously associated with homosexuality, although it sometimes tends to be associated with it. In this condition the afflicted person more or less

identifies himself (or herself) with the opposite sex, not only in dress but in general tastes, in ways of acting, and in emotional disposition. The problem of transvestism is an extremely difficult one, and there seems to be two lines of thought:[24]

1) that it is consequent upon early psychological experiences —this is favored by the majority of psychiatrists.
2) that it is constitutional—this seems to be favored by the endocrinologists.

(2) The author feels that testicular biopsies are essential as part of the diagnostic as well as therapeutic armentarium in the management of cases of transvestism. Where the arrest of spermatogenesis and/or atrophic changes in the seminiferous tubules can be demonstrated, the biologic factors cannot be denied.

(3) Since the disorder may manifest itself as early as the fourth or fifth year, the physician should be alerted to the early detection or tendency toward transvestism.

REFERENCES

1. Hirschfeld, M.: *Sexual Anomalies and Perversions.* F. Adler, London, 1936.
2. Krafft-Ebing, R. nov.: *Psychopathia Sexualis.* Pioneer Publications, New York, 1947.
3. Stekel, W.: *Impotence in the Male.* Vol. 1 and 2. Translation by Bolz, H. O. London, John Lane, The Bodley Head, Ltd., 1955.
4. Armstrong, N. C.: Transvestism. In Symposium on *Nuclear Sex,* edited by Smith, R. D., and Davidson, M. W. Interscience Publishers, Inc., New York, 1958.
5. Lukianowicz, N.: Survey of various aspects of transvestism in the light of our present knowledge. *J. of New and Mental Disease, 128:* 36-61, 1959.
6. Barr, M. L., and Hobbs, G. E.: Chromosomal sex in transvestites. *Lancet, 1:* 1109-1110, 1954.
7. Moore, K. L., and Barr, M. L.: Morphology of nerve cell nucleus in mammals with special reference to sex chromatin. *J. Comp. Neurol., 98:* 213-231, 1953.
8. Moore, K. L., and Barr, M. L.: Smears from the oral mucosa in the detection of chromosomal sex. *Lancet, 2:* 57-8, 1955.
9. Moore, K. L., Graham, M. A., and Barr, M. L.: Detection of chromosomal sex in hermaphrodites from a skin biopsy. *Surg. Gynec. & Obst., 96:* 641-648, 1953.

10. Klinefelter, H. F.: Klinefelter's Syndrome in: Jones, H. W., and Scott, W. W.: *Hermaphroditism, Genital Anomalies and Related Endocrine Disorders,* Chapter VI, Williams and Wilkins, Baltimore, 1958.
11. Klinefelter, H. F., Reifenstein, E. C., and Albright, F.: Syndrome characterized by gynecomastia, aspermatogenesis with aleydigism and increased excretion of follicle stimulating hormone. *J. Clin. Endocrinol., 2:* 615, 1942.
12. Davidson, W. M., and Smith, R. D.: The Neutrophil sex nodules in Klinefelter's Syndrome. Symposium on *Nuclear Sex,* p. 93, William Heinman Medical Books, Ltd., London.
13. Grumbach, M.: Special Article. The sex chromatin pattern and human sexual anomalies. *Year Book of Endocrinology,* 1959-1959, p. 281, Year Book Publishers, Chicago.
14. Randell, J. B.: Transvestism and trans-sexualism—a study of 50 cases. *Brit. M. J., 1448:* Dec. 26, 1959.
15. Warden, L., and Marsh, N. N. Quoted by Lukianowicz, N. Survey of various aspects of transvestism in the light of our present knowledge. *J. of Nev. and Mental Disease, 128:* 36-61, 1959.
16. Bak, R. C.: Fetishism. *A. Am. Psychoanalyt. A., 1:* 289-294, 1953.
17. Greene, R.: In discussion after presentation of: Transvestism. Armstrong, N. C. In *Symposium on Nuclear Sex,* edited by Smith, R. D. and Davidson, M. W. Interscience Publishers, Inc., New York, 1958.
18. Siebenmann, E. R.: In discussion after presentation of: Transvestism. Armstrong, N. C. In *Symposium on Nuclear Sex,* edited by Smith, R. D., and Davidson, M. W. Interscience Publishers, Inc., New York, 1958.
19. Davidson, M. W.: In discussion after presentation of: Transvestism. Armstrong, N. C. In *Symposium on Nuclear Sex,* edited by Smith, R. D., and Davidson, M. W. Interscience Publishers, Inc., New York, 1958.
20. Bishop, P. M. F.: In discussion after presentation of: Transvestism. Armstrong, N. C. In Symposium on Nuclear Sex, edited by Smith, R. D., and Davidson, M. W. Interscience Publishers, Inc., New York, 1958.
21. Bakwin, H.: Transvestism in children. *J. Ped., 56:* 294, 1960.
22. Ellis, H.: Eonism and other Studies: In *Studies in the Psychology of Sex,* Vol. 2, Random House, New York, 1936.
23. Oliven, F. J.: Sexual Hygiene and Pathology. Chapter 21. *Sexual Deviations.* J. B. Lippincott Co., Philadelphia and Montreal, 1955.
24. Armstrong, N. C.: Personal communication.
25. Wilkins, L.: *The Diagnosis and Treatment of Endocrine Disorders in Childhood and Adolescence.* Thomas, Springfield, 2nd ed., 1957.

Chapter 14

TESTIS IN THE AGED

JUST AS ONE must consider and evaluate growth and development of the testis, so one must consider and evaluate aging of the testis. Biologic criteria of the process of aging are few, scattered, and in many instances, equivocal.[1] This is not surprising, since the mechanism of testicular function in this age group is poorly understood. Considerable data exists on testicular embryology, hormonal influences and pre-puberal, puberal and post-puberal testicular morphology and function, yet the true morphology and function of the senescent testis, remains at this time, obscure.

The reader will recall that in the chapter on spermatogenesis, attention was directed to the striking difference between oogenesis in the female and spermatogenesis in the male. It was pointed out that the aging process in the male gonad, is not as marked or uniform as it is in the chronological years of aging in the female gonad. In the male, it is a variable factor and differs markedly in individuals.

Engle[2,3] believes that this difference is so marked, that it is proper to compare the two processes, thereby gaining some insight from the comparison. To quote Engle, "The human gonads, the ovary and the testis, have two attributes in common. Both secrete steroids, not necessarily specific to them, and they both elaborate germ cells which are specific to them. There the comparison ends. The entire life history of the human ovary is dominated by the egg: the ovum. When the eggs are all gone the ovary, normally, is an inert residue of connective tissue. The several metabolic functions of the testes are apparently completely independent of its gametogenic function. In the female the ovarian steroids are normally produced only under the influence of the egg. In the male the elaboration of testicular steroids is completely independent of sperm production. In the female the menopause occurs in a specific age range because the eggs are gone. In the male there is no abrupt cessation of testicular endrogens. The decline in the output of 17-ketosteroids is gradual and has great individual variation. This is the reason that symptoms of the climacteric are seen in about one third of women but are very rare in men."

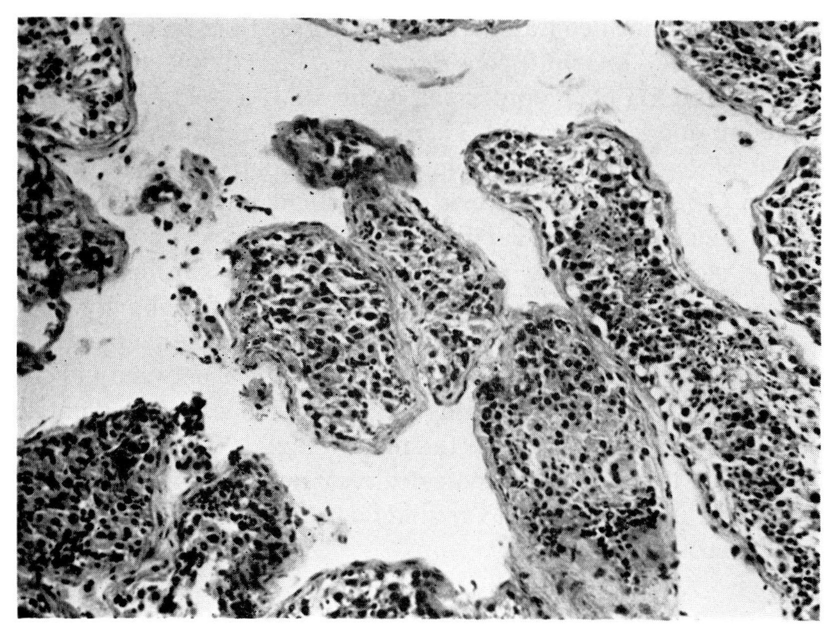

FIG. 35. Photomicrograph of section of testicle removed from white male, age 69, because of carcinoma of prostate. Note minimal degenerative and atrophic changes in tubules. Spermatids in moderate numbers, germinal epithelium intact and still active—some mitotic figures.

This does not mean that degeneration of the seminiferous tubules does not occur in aged men. It does occur and in such cases it is believed that degenerative changes, especially of the blood vessels, prohibits sperm production. Of singular interest is that when pathologic processes do occur in the testes of the aged it is characterized by a *thickening of the basement membrane* and the presence of *small round cells* instead of spermatogenic cells. This histologic picture is similar to that seen in undeveloped testes of young males.

On the other hand the histologic picture of the testes of the aged dying from accidental death is not essentially different from that of younger men. The author has on several occasions taken

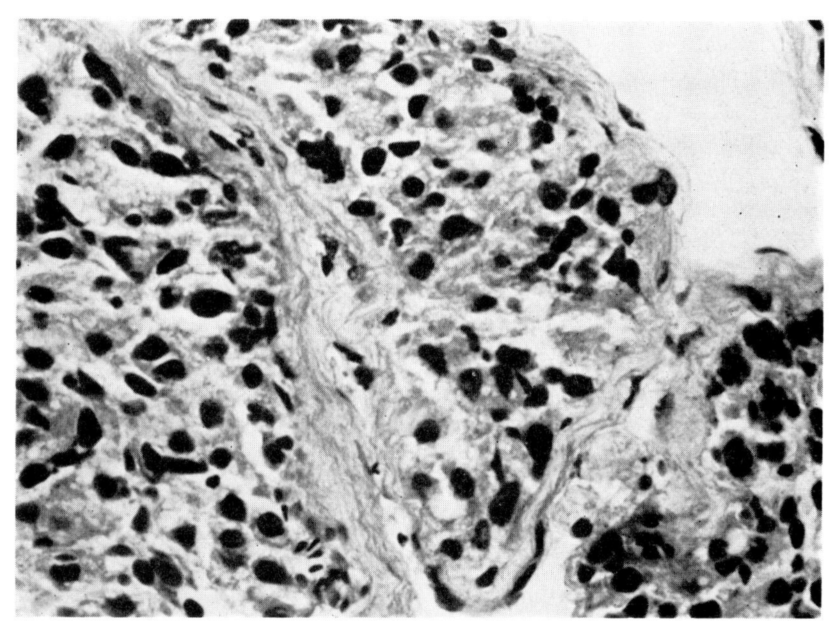

FIG. 36. Photomicrograph of section of testicle—high power—same case as Figure 35. Note comparatively thin basement membrane.

biopsies while performing prostatectomies in elderly males (80-90 years of age) and has been amazed at the most orderly and normal histological testicular architecture. Despite such findings it is difficult to make positive statements about the testis of the aged person because of the many variations.

Since spermatogenesis is one of the important functions of the testis it would be most appropriate to determine whether this function of the testis is altered with age. Hypospermatogenesis does occur in the aged (as well as in the young) but the exact mechanism is not entirely understood. When spermatogenesis is

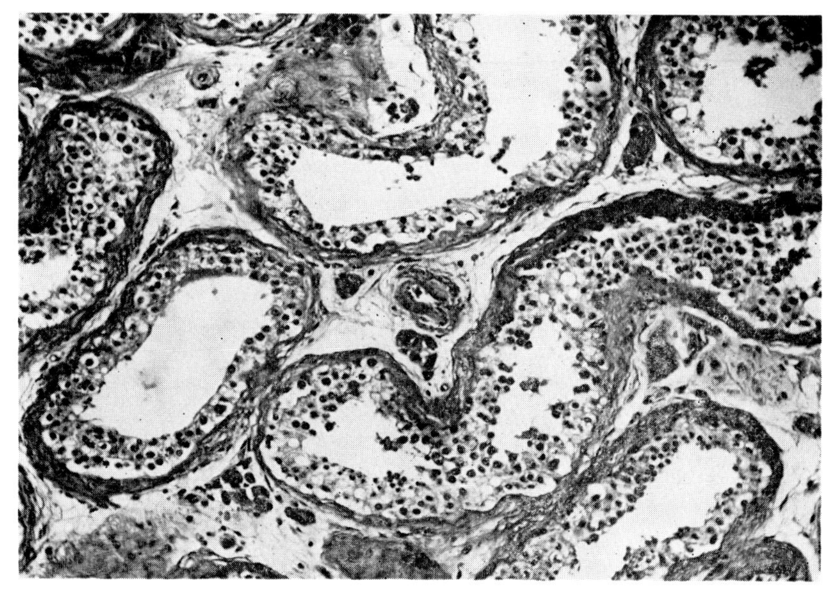

FIG. 37. Photomicrograph of section of testicle removed from white male, age 72, because of carcinoma of prostate. Note normal architectural pattern with minimal degenerative and atrophic changes in tubules.

arrested, it seems to occur most frequently at the primary spermatocyte stage. This has been described by Sniffen[4] in the following manner: "The lowering of spermatogenic activity and the consequent decrease in the number of lumen cells make the tubule seem dilated; the outside diameter of the tubule is unaltered, however. In the event of complete spermatogenic failure the Sertoli cells gradually become atrophic, but first they show a moderate number of large sudanophilic globules in their cytoplasm." At this time certain changes take place in the wall of the seminiferous tubule all of which are difficult to interpret. Many believe that the most marked change is that of definite thickening of the basement membrane. Engle[5] believes that this change in the basement membrane and the capsule of the tubule (tunica propria) is most significant in failing spermatogenic activity. "Normally," states Engle, "this is a delicate basement membrane which is surrounded by laminated collagenous and argyophile fibers. In all tubules of man or monkey during the ages of sperm formation, this is a thin and delicate membrane if the tubules are in normal spermatogenic condition. The connective tissue of the tunica propria increases in thickness in many individuals, usually with decrease in the size of the tubule." Progressive changes occur with ultimate closure of the lumen and production of tubular sclerosis and disappearance of the Sertoli cells due to compression. Thus there occurs a rapid thickening of the basement membrane so the germ cells die and are replaced by connective tissue. We do not know why this occurs and what institutes the process and as yet this change in the basement membrane of the tubules has never been experimentally produced in animals.*

What is confusing in a study of the testis of the elderly man, is that there is often no change in the interstitial cells. In fact in many elderly persons the interstitial cells are similar cytologically to those of a young man. Sniffen[4] has described a common distortion, which is not encountered in young men. The Leydig cells take the form of small compact groups, lying in angles between the tubules, isolated by wide intervals from each other without the intervention, between the groups, of other Leydig cells.

As stated previously, the testis of the aged is often associated with a thickened basement membrane. When this occurs the spermatogenic cells change into small round cells and the histologic picture then closely resembles the testicular histology seen in the undeveloped testis of the young male. Such changes are purely involutional and can be seen in the testis of the hypophysectomized adult male monkey. When the pituitary gland is removed in such an animal, the spermatogenic cell undergo a prompt dedifferentiation and, in the terminal stage, show all of the histological characters of the undifferentiated epithelium of the pre-puberal resting testis.

---

*It is well established that the first evidence of puberty in the testis is the formation of the tubular tunica propria. In the absence of male sex hormone activity this structure never forms, as is the case in hypergonadotropic eunuchoids even in the fourth and fifth decades of life. When one sees evidence of the tunica propria being deposited in young boys, one can predict rather confidently that within the next year or so other evidences of puberty will be manifested. It certainly represents activity of the Leydig cells prior to germinal cell activity.

Stieve[6] believes the tubules in the aged retain the same approximate width when sperm bearing, and have no more involutionary changes than those seen in the young men, providing no serious medical complication exists. This author believes the tubules of the aged not to be round but angled. This, Engle[5] thought might be the result of increase in elastic fibers and decrease of collagenous fibers in the tubule wall. It would seem to the writer that it would more logically be the result of a decrease in elastic fibers in the tubule wall associated with similar changes elsewhere in the anatomical structure of the elderly person.

The changes seen in the atrophic senile testis may also be seen in younger men. Such changes occur when the testis has been injured by general illness, trauma or disease. Chronic illnesses present at puberty retard the differentiation and normal development of the testis. "A lag in maturation regularly occurs in the presence of fever and infection, but these conditions are prerequisites. For example, in congenital heart disease with circulatory failure, the tubules may fail to mature by the late teens and sclerosis of the tunica propria may develop . . . In some adolescent boys who have died of chronic illness, not only is there retardation of tubular development, but occasionally the Sertoli cells show degenerative changes in the form of coarse eosinophilic granules in the cytoplasm with distintegration of the cells. In addition, the Leydig cells do not develop at the expected time and the interstitial tissue appears to contain only 'fibroblasts.'[7]

The role of the interstitial cells in the senile testis has always received great attention but as yet no definite relation between these cells and sexual activity has been established. The major function of the testicular tubule is sperm production but it has been speculated that the tubular cells may also play a role in the production of hormones. Androgen is the most active hormone and this arises from testosterone manufactured in the Leydig cell. Other hormones are also present in the testicle. Estrogen is present in the testis of the bull, and the stallion, and estradiol has been extracted from the human testis. Maddock[8] and Nelson believe this hormone may arise from the Leydig cells, "since increase in urinary estrogen have been demonstrated in men who have

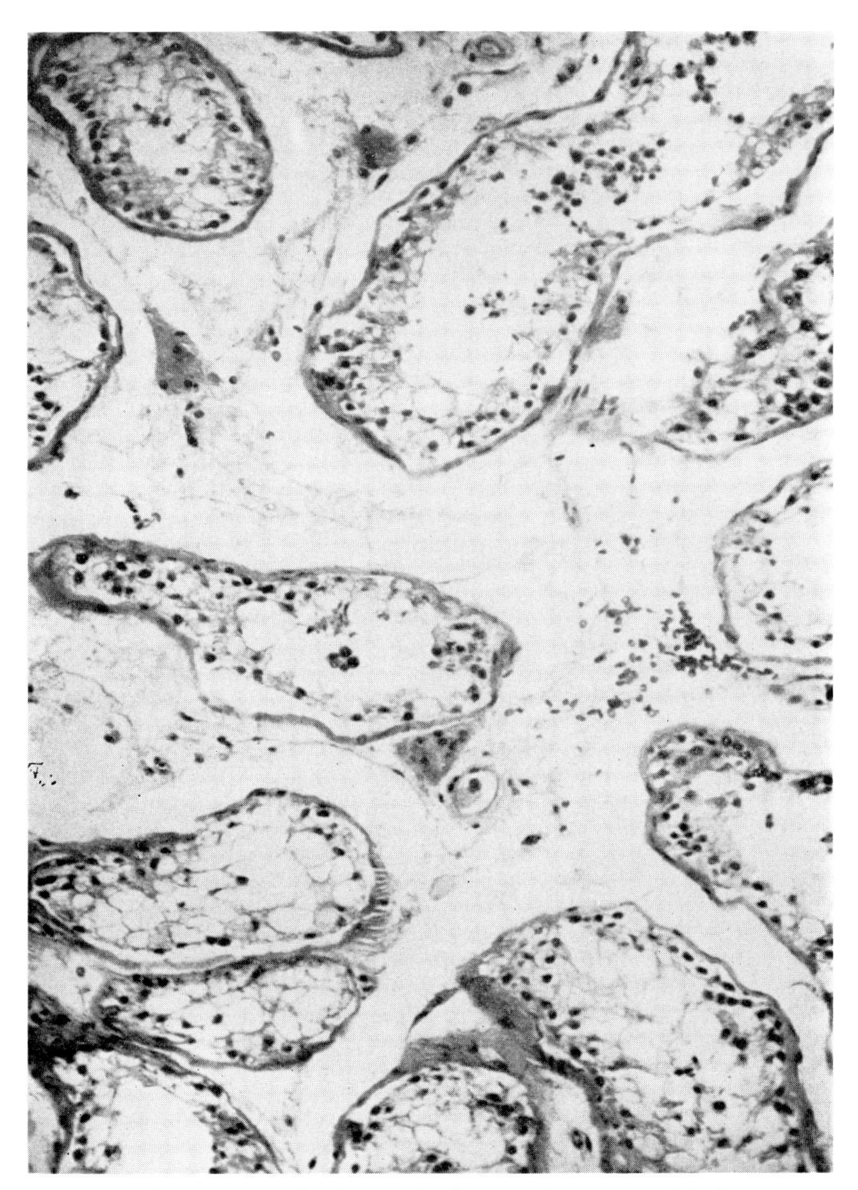

FIG. 38. Photomicrograph of testicular biopsy of negro age 90, demonstrating degeneration and partial atrophy of germinal epitheluim. Spermatogenesis is reduced but present.

received chorionic gonadotropin injections, and this is associated with an increase in the number of Leydig cells without change in Sertoli cells and a decrease in spermatogenesis." Others believe that the Sertoli cells are the source of testicular estrogen. That this may be the case is strongly suggested by the feminization which is seen in Sertoli cell tumors in dogs and in the human.[9,10,11] McCullough[12] and Schaffenburg also cite the work in which pragneolone has also been shown to be present in the testis.[13] Since this substance under experimental conditions stimulates gametogenesis or manifests it in the absence of the hyphophysis certain hormonal speculation appears more logical, and the belief that hormones arise in tubular epithelium may be of great significance in the future evaluation of the senile testis. Significantly, chorionic gonadotropin injections, in hypogonadotropic eunuchoids and in relatively normal men produces tubular activity and in some instances at least partial spermatogenesis; whereas if spermatogenesis is established, such therapy produces spermatogenic damage. Nelson[8] and Maddock interpret this as occurring because of increased output of androgens and estrogens which inhibit pituitary FSH and thereby interfere with normal spermatogenesis.

The reader must recall that the Sertoli cells are the first testicular cells to differentiate in the embryo, and significantly they are the last to disappear in old age. The Sertoli cells differ from other cells. Little is known about the internal chemistry of the Sertoli cell but it is accepted that its presence within the tubule is essential for the maturation of the sperm cell. The Sertoli cell is atypical in that it has no apical membrane. It has a free-flowing colloidal cytoplasm at the apex, which is moving and changing within the tubule. As sperm develop and the spermatid is formed and begins to go through the normal process of growth, it is taken up and nurtured by the Sertoli cell.

The Leydig cell on the other hand has little if any relation to gametogenesis. It can produce hormones independently of the presence of sperm. Thus young males with complete fibrosis of the seminiferous tubules may have normal genital development, normal sexual activity and normal production of 17-ketosteroids.

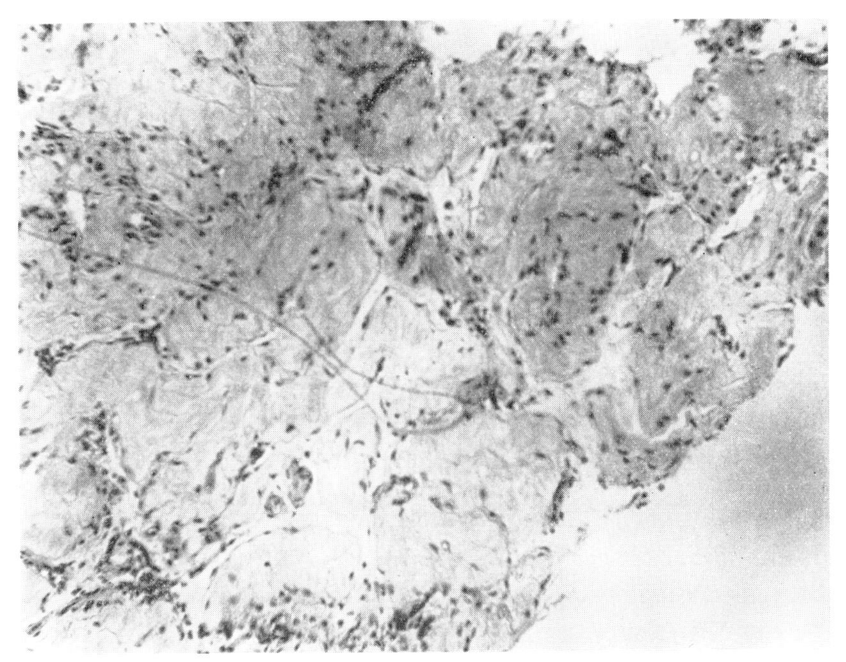

FIG. 39. Photomicrograph of testicular biopsy, of colored male, age 85, with long history of chronic systemic diseases. Note hyalinization of seminiferous tubules and thickness of basement membrane.

The male has an entirely separate unit for hormone production, whereas in the female, hormone production is dependent upon successive development of a series of follicle bearing eggs.

Despite the realization that hormones may stimulate development in youth, there is no evidence that their administration retards the tendency to senescence.[28] It was the hope of earlier workers that a knowledge of the endocrine function and the subsequent availability of hormones, that the hoped for "fountain of perpetual youth" would be materialized. Indeed it can be said that although the endocrine glands age as do all tissues and organs, there is no evidence that a particular tendency for these to deteriorate is associated with the ageing process.

Most articles dealing with the senile testis make reference to pigment and granules in the Leydig cells. Sniffen,[4] Engle[5] and others,[14, 15] do not believe that the presence of pigment is significant of senescent, although seen in many males beyond 60 years of age. It is to be hoped that localization of specific substances as pigment granules by cytochemical methods will ultimately clarify this phase of the senescent testis. Some measures of the significance of cytochemical studies is well demonstrated in the work of Lynch,[16] Scott,[17] Engle,[2, 3, 5, 18] Long[19] and Montagna. Cytological observations on the human testis continue to help assemble a definite pattern. Thus Lynch[17] and Scott in careful studies of the human and animal testis deduced the following information regarding the lipid produced in the Sertoli cell: The lipid does not appear until puberty and then only after the appearance of lipid in the Leydig cell. This supports the belief that both androgen from the Leydig cells and follicle stimulating hormone from the pituitary are required for proper function of the seminiferous tubules. Mature spermatogenesis appears simultaneously with demonstrable Sertoli cell lipid indicating that the lipid is necessary for the production of spermatozoa. The lipid is released into the lumina of the tubules with the mature sperm, but retained within the Sertoli cells in the absence of spermatogenesis. This is compatible with the hypothesis that the Sertoli cells have a nutritive function and suggests that the lipid may well be the nutritive material."

Nelson[21] believes this picture seen in the Sertoli cell is universally proportional to the activity of the germinal epithelium and is seen after hypophysectomy, estrogen treatment, cryptorchidism, x-ray-irradiated testes, testes of animals receiving androgens in which spermatogenesis is interfered with and in the testes of animals receiving nitrofuranes. Nelson has also seen this condition in the testes of men who have suffered severe febrile episodes that caused cessation of spermatogenesis. Thus after pneumonia a cessation of spermatogenesis continues for some time. In the senile testis, with less active spermatogenesis, an accumulation of lipid in the Sertoli cells can be demonstrated and probably is indicative of decline in spermatogenesis.

THE MALE CLIMACTERIC

The end of reproductive life in the female is a gonadal process, extending over a period of one to three years and usually at some time between the ages of 45 and 50. The term climacteric (meaning rung of a ladder) is preferred to the use of the word menopause, which truly refers to a cessation of menstruation. The same term has also been used in regard to the male with signs and symptoms of the supposed 'male menopause.' It would indeed be more logical to refer to such changes in the male as the male climacteric, even though many doubt such a state of affairs exist in the male.

One thing is certain about the termination of reproductive life in the male as compared to the female; it is more gradual and more variable in men than in women. Indeed many men never pass through a physiological readjustment comparable with the female climacteric. Some men, however, appear to suffer the same symptoms and to show the same rise in the level of gonadotropin excretion as those described in the case of women.[22] The majority of men, however, enter into a period of sexual decline in a most gradual manner and without producing clinical signs.

Segal[23] and Nelson in evaluating testicular function in aging males analyzed various hormone excretion levels of men, ranging in age to nearly 100 years. The trend in the average 17-ketosteroid excretions with advancing decades of life reveals a gradual decline, until 60 years of age, but the value remains relatively constant thereafter. In addition to 17-ketosteroid excretion, gonadotropin study and estrogenic studies wherever feasable were made. Of singular interest was that testicular biopsies were taken from most individuals for whom the urinary excretion patterns were determined. Segal and Nelson's observations are as follows: The trend in the average 17-ketosteroids with advancing decades of life, showed a gradual decline with aging until 60 years, but the value remains relatively constant thereafter. The normal range for young reproductive males is established as 6.0 mg. to 10.0 mg. per 24 hours. Until age 60, the average, though declining remains in the normal range. Even among octogenarians, these workers found individuals with urinary 17-ketosteroid values within range for normal, young adults.*

---

*Determinations of 17-ketosteroid excretion values were carried out on three consecutive 24-hour urine samples from each subject, using the Zimmerman reaction following acid hydrolysis. Corrections were based on creatinine determinations.

The percentage of cases with elevated gonadotropins increased only slightly with aging. But increased gonadotropin excretion was not even generally characteristic of old age in the male. In the oldest age group, more than 50% of the cases had average excretion values.*

The estrogen excretion values were at non-assayable levels in approximately 10% of the cases in the oldest age group, while elevated levels occurred in almost 40%. The remaining 50% retained average excretion values.**

Testicular biopsies in about 20% of the cases showed active spermatogenesis slight to moderate fibrosis and Leydig cells. Most showed an essentially normal testicular histology. The largest percentage of biopsies revealed progressing fibrosis, poor to active spermatogenesis, and Leydig cells which appeared active by histologic anatomy.

Heller and Myers[24] studied 23 men with vasomotor symptoms, as well as psychic, sexual and urinary symptoms suggestive of male climacteric. All had increase of urinary excretion of gonadotropins. Testicular biopsies in eight cases revealed abnormal Leydig cells, with a decrease in size and activity of the seminiferous tubules. Howard *et al.*,[25] in a study of six patients were unable to confirm the presence of abnormal testicular histology. The author[26] has performed similiar study in 25 patients, in which only few (3) cases revealed hyalinization (as seen in Klinefelter's syndrome) and the remainder revealed normal Leydig cells, normal seminiferous tubules and evidence of gametogenesis.

Sohval[27] advises the therapeutic test of 25 mg. of testosterone propionate, to be given intramuscularly 5 times a week for two weeks. "A lack of response practically excludes the diagnosis of male climacteric and identifies the symptoms as psychogenic. On

---

*Evaluation of total urinary gonadotropins were determined by these authors, by biological assay, following kaolin extraction of three consecutive 24-hour urine specimens from each subject. Assays were evaluated on uterine weight increase in immature female mice.

**These authors assayed biologically urinary estrogens using the phenolic fraction recovered after NaOH extraction of three consecutive 24-hour urine specimens from each subject. Assays were evaluated on uterine weight increase in immature female rats.

the other hand, a beneficial result may be due to the effects of suggestion to which psychoneurotic patients are often susceptible. Where this is suspected the course of treatment should be repeated using plain seasame oil instead. A continued good response will confirm this suspicion." Sohval advises to first determine that no contraindications to androgen administration exist. Digital rectal examination should be utilized to exclude the possibility of carcinoma of the prostate which would be aggravated by androgens.

It is the author's opinion that there is no definite male climacteric. It is true that certain symptoms may appear in the senescent male but these symptoms are not necessarily those of a climacteric similiar to the change seen in aging women. Since the decline as pointed out by Engle and others in the output of 17-ketosteroids in the older male is gradual and has great individual variation it is more logical to assume that an abrupt hormonal change such as seen in the female can occur in the male. Further as pointed out by most workers in this field the only morphological characteristics of the senescent testicle is the progressively increased amount of tubular fibrosis. Although this fibrosis parallels the climb of androgen production we still do not know which is effect and which is cause.

SUMMARY

(1) The male gonad continues to function late in life, and differs markedly in this respect from the female gonad.

(2) What determines the difference from a consideration of senescence between the male and the female germ cells is unknown.

(3) The Sertoli cells which undoubtedly hold the key to the solution of this problem are the first testicular cells to differentiate in the embryo, and they are the last to disappear in old age.

(4) In the male (in contrast to the female) the elaboration of testicular steroids is completely independent of sperm production. Ovarian steroids are normally produced only under the influence of the ovum.

(5) Testicular changes in the aged are not necessarily associated with so-called "climacteric" symptoms.

REFERENCES

1. Magladery, J. W.: Neurophysiology of Aging's. In Birren, J. E., editor. *Handbook of Aging and the Individual,* p. 173, University of Chicago Press, Chicago, Ill., 1959.
2. Engle, E. T.: In Conference on Problems of Aging. Sponsored by Josiah Macy Jr. Foundation: Endocrine Aspects of Aging, New York, 1951.
3. Engle, E. T.: The life history of the human testis. *J. Urol., 74:* 379, p. 379-385, 1958.
4. Sniffen, R. C.: The Testis. 1. The normal testis. *Arch. of Pathology,* Vol. 50, No. 3, p. 281, Sept. 1950.
5. Engle, E. T.: The testis and hormones. Chapter 17. In Cowdry, E. V., editor: *Problems of Aging.* Williams & Wilkins Co., Baltimore, 1942.
6. Stieve, H.: Mannliche Genitalorgane. In von Mollendorf, *Handbuch der Mikro. Anat. der Menschen,* V 11-2, 11, 1930.
7. Sniffen, R. C.: Histology of the normal and abnormal testis at puberty. *Ann. of New York Acad. of Sc., 55:* 613, 1952.
8. Maddock, W. O., and Nelson, W. O.: Increased estrogen excretion due to stimulation of Leydig cells in adult men receiving chorionic gonadotropin. Assoc. Study Internal Secretions, 33rd meeting, Atlantic City, N. J., 1951.
9. Huggins, C., and Moulder, P. V.: Estrogen production by Sertoli cell tumors of testis. *Cancer Research, 5:* 510, 1945.
10. Berthrong, M., Goodwin, W. E., and Scott, W. W.: Estrogen production by testis. *J. Clin. Endocrinol., 9:* 579, 1949.
11. Teilum, G.: Estrogen-producing Sertoli cell tumors (androblastoma tubulare lipoides) of human testis and ovary. Homologous ovarian and testicular tumors. 111. *J. Clin. Endocrinol., 9:* 579, 1949.
12. McCullagh, E. P., and Schaffenburg, C. A.: The role of the seminiferous tubules in the production of hormones. *Ann. New York Acad. Sc., 55:* 674, 1952.
13. Haines, W. J., Johnson, R. H., et al.: Biochemical studies on hog testicular extract. 1. Isolation and identification of 5-pregnen-3-B-ol-20-one. *J. Biol. Chem., 174:* 925, 1948.
14. Montagna, W., and Hamilton, J. B.: Histological studies of human testes. 1. The distribution of lipids. *Anat. Record., 109:* 635-660, 1951.
15. Montagna, W., and Hamilton, J. B.: Histological studies of human testes. 2. The distribution of glycogen and other $H\ 10_4$ Schiff reactive substances. *Anat. Record., 112:* 237-250, 1952.
16. Lynch, K. M.: Recovery of the rat testis following estrogen therapy. *Ann. of New York Acad. Sc., 55:* 734, 1952.

17. Lynch, K. M., and Scott, W. W.: The lipoid content of the Leydig cell and Sertoli cell in the human testis as related to age, benign prostatic hyperplasia and prostatic cancer. *J. Urol., 64:* 767, 1950.
18. Long, M. E., and Engle, E. T.: Cytochemistry of the human testis. *Ann. of New York Acad. Sc., 55:* 619, 1952.
19. Long, M. E., Quoted by Engle, E. T.: In Conference on Problems of Aging. Sponsored by Josiah Macy Jr. Foundation: Endocrine Aspects of Aging. New York, 1951.
20. Montagna, W.: Some cytochemical observations on the human testes and epididymides. *Ann. New York Acad. Sc., 55:* 629, 1952.
21. Nelson, W. O.: Sex differences in human nuclei with particular reference to the ketosteroid gonad agenesis and other types of hermaphrodites. *Acta Endocrinol., 23:* 227-245, 1956.
22. Hall, P. F.: *The Functions of the Endocrine Glands.* W. B. Saunders Co., Philadelphia, p. 249, 1959.
23. Segal, S. J., Nelson, W. O.: Initiation and maintenance of testicular function. *Conference on Recent Progress in the Endocrinology of Reproduction.* Lloyd, C. W., editor. Academic Press Inc., New York and London, 1959.
24. Heller, G. G., and Myers, G. B.: Male Climacteric. *J.A.M.A., 126:* 472, 1944.
25. Howard, R. P., Sniffen, R. C., Simons, F. A., and Albright, F.: Testicular Deficiency. *J. Clin. Endocrinol., 10:* 121, 1950.
26. Wershub, L. P.: Testicular biopsy in the aged. To be published.
27. Sohval, A. R.: Diseases of the testis. Chapter 17. In Soffer, L. J.: *Diseases of the Endocrine Glands.* Second edition, p. 524, Lea and Febiger, Philadelphia, 1956.
28. Grollman, A.: *Disorders of the Endocrine System in the Older Patient.* Ed. Johnson, N. W., Paul B. Hoeber, Inc., New York, 1960.

AUTHOR INDEX

Y

Z

SUBJECT INDEX

B

D

E

F

G

H

I

T

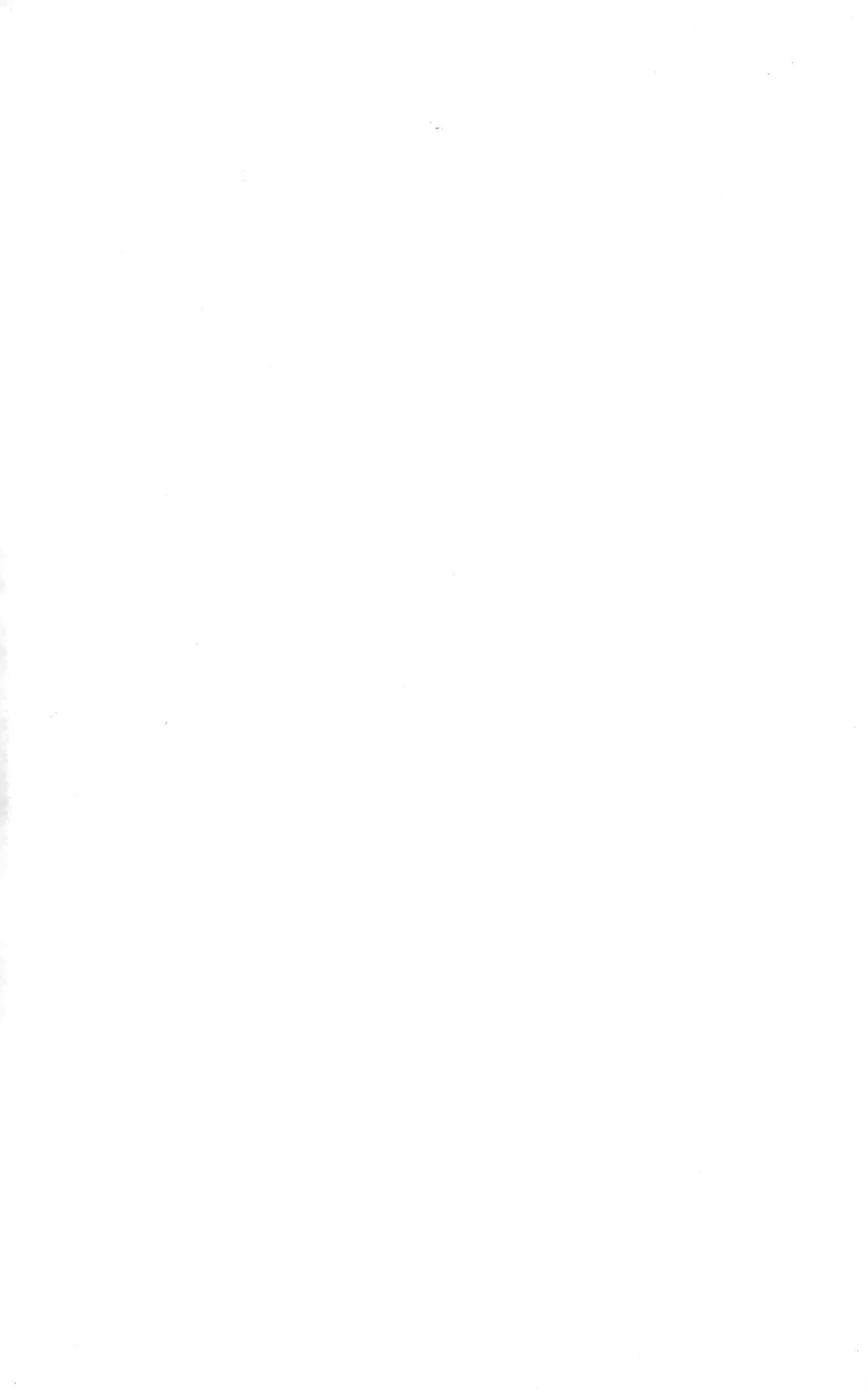

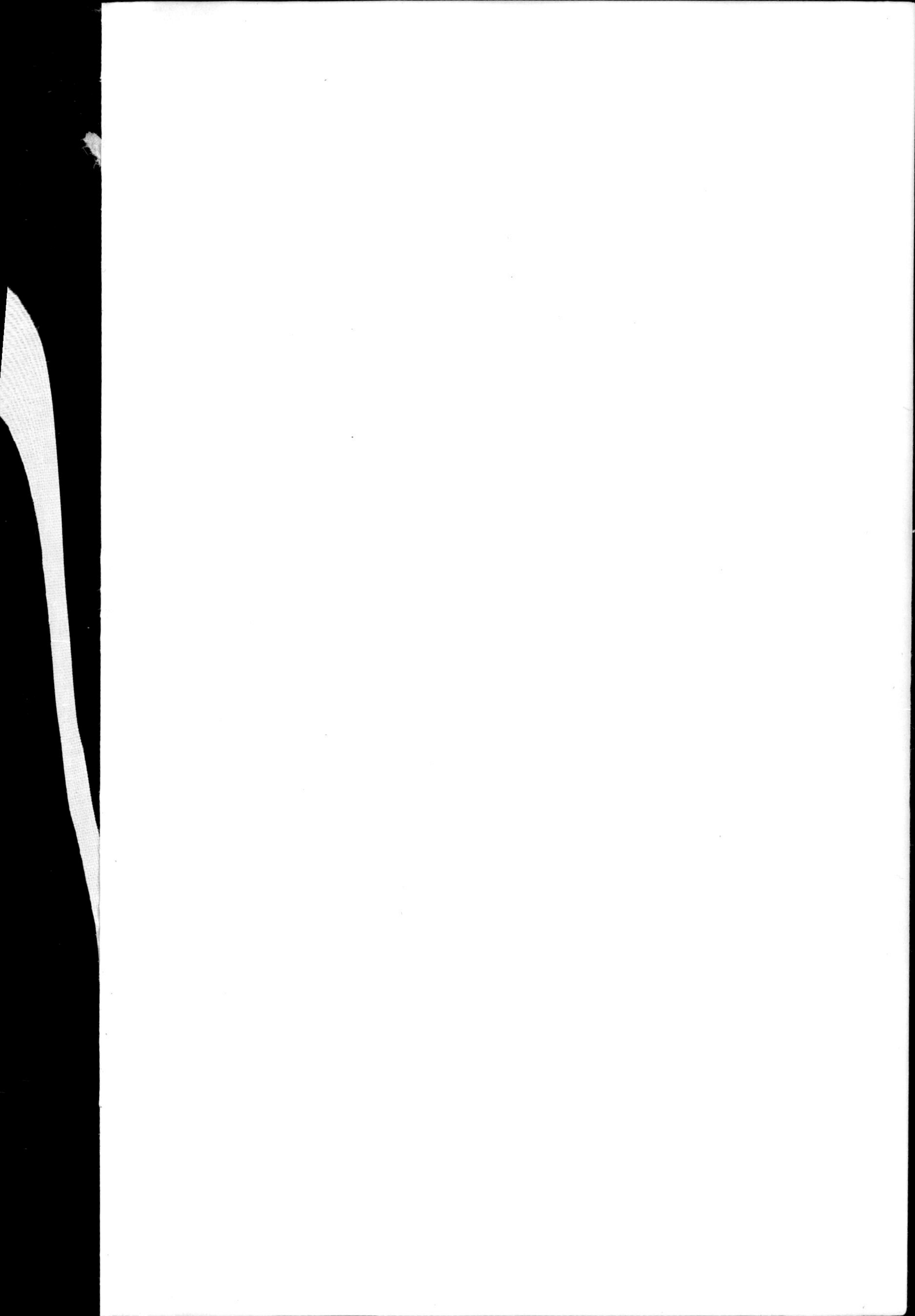